Ethnicity, Health, and Primary Care

Edited by

Joe Kai
Division of Primary Care
School of Community Health Sciences
University of Nottingham

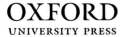

OXFORD
UNIVERSITY PRESS

*This book has been printed digitally and produced in a standard specification
in order to ensure its continuing availability*

OXFORD
UNIVERSITY PRESS

Great Clarendon Street, Oxford OX2 6DP

Oxford University Press is a department of the University of Oxford.
It furthers the University's objective of excellence in research, scholarship,
and education by publishing worldwide in

Oxford New York

Auckland Cape Town Dar es Salaam Hong Kong Karachi
Kuala Lumpur Madrid Melbourne Mexico City Nairobi
New Delhi Shanghai Taipei Toronto
With offices in
Argentina Austria Brazil Chile Czech Republic France Greece
Guatemala Hungary Italy Japan South Korea Poland Portugal
Singapore Switzerland Thailand Turkey Ukraine Vietnam

Oxford is a registered trade mark of Oxford University Press
in the UK and in certain other countries

Published in the United States
by Oxford University Press Inc., New York

© Oxford University Press 2003

The moral rights of the author have been asserted

Database right Oxford University Press (maker)

Reprinted 2006

ISBN 0-19-851573-1

Acknowledgements

The publishers and editor thank the following for permission to reproduce or modify copyright material:

The Office for National Statistics for Table 1.2.
BMJ Publishing Group for Table 2.1 and Chapter 17.1.
Medical Education for Box 10.1.

The Royal College of General Practitioners for permission to reproduce the illustration in Box 10.2.

The Health Development Agency for permission to reproduce Table 19.1, from *Sickle Cell and Thalassaemia: Achieving Health Gain. Guidance for Commissioners and Providers*, © Queen's Printer and Controller of HMSO.

I am grateful indeed to all the contributors for generously producing fine chapters despite their many other commitments, and for graciously accommodating editorial suggestions or interference. I have enjoyed the support of many other friends and colleagues, and particularly thank Philippa Matthews, and the University of Birmingham where I developed some of this volume. Finally I thank Sophia Christie, Chief Executive of Eastern Birmingham Primary Care Trust, for helpful discussion about addressing racism in health care practice.

Joe Kai

Contents

Contributors

Akgul Baylav has been active developing community health advocacy for many years in London. She works as Equalities Adviser at Barking & Dagenham Primary Care Trust.

Raj Bhopal holds the Alexander Bruce and John Usher Chair of Public Health at the University of Edinburgh, is head of the Division of Community Health Sciences, and is honorary consultant in public health medicine at the Lothian Health Board.

Angela Burnett is a general practitioner who is currently developing the Sanctuary Practice for newly arrived asylum seekers and refugees in Hackney, East London. She also works at the Medical Foundation for the Care of Victims of Torture.

Lai Fong Chiu has a background in community work and health promotion, developing the 'Community Health Educator' model in the UK. She is now a Senior Research Fellow at the Nuffield Institute for Health, University of Leeds.

Christina Faull has been a Consultant in Palliative Care working in hospital, hospice and community settings based at University Hospital Birmingham. Recently she has developed a community palliative care advocacy service to enhance the care of people from diverse ethnic communities with advanced cancer.

Azhar Farooqi is a general practitioner working with a multi-ethnic population in central Leicester, and Honorary Senior Lecturer in the Department of General Practice and Primary Care at University of Leicester.

Jon Fuller has been a general practitioner in Hackney since 1979 and developed a course for bilingual health advocates in East London with Akgul Baylav. He is Head of the Graduate Entry Medical Programme at St Bartholomew's and the London Hospital at Queen Mary College, University of London.

Katy Gardner is an inner-city general practitioner at Princes Park Health Centre in Liverpool with a special interest in community involvement and inequalities in access to health care. She has been involved in 'ethnicity monitoring', more recently patient profiling, for 10 years.

Abdul Rashid Gatrad is a consultant pediatrician at Manor Hospital in Walsall, Honorary Senior Lecturer at the University of Birmingham and Honorary Assistant Professor at the University of Kentucky, USA.

Paramjit Gill is an inner-city general practitioner in Birmingham and Senior Lecturer in Primary Care at the University of Birmingham.

Louise Hammersley has been an inner-city general practitioner in

Birmingham and now works in Lichfield.

Steve Iliffe has been a general practitioner in Kilburn, north-west London, since 1978. He is Reader in General Practice at the Royal Free and UCL Medical School, and co-director of the Centre for Ageing Population Studies there.

Mark R. D. Johnson is Professor of Diversity in Health & Social Care at De Montfort University. He directs the Centre for Evidence in Ethnicity Health and Diversity at the Mary Seacole Research Centre in Leicester.

Ben Jones works in primary care with Central Liverpool Primary Care Trust. He enjoys his work, and his work enjoys him.

David Jones works as a general practitioner on the Broadwater Farm Estate in Tottenham, North London. He is a Lecturer in the Department of Primary Care Primary Care and Population Sciences at the Royal Free Hospital and University College London School of Medicine.

Joe Kai has been an inner-city general practitioner and primary care academic in both Newcastle upon Tyne and Birmingham. He is Professor of Primary Care in the School of Community Health Sciences, University of Nottingham.

Kamlesh Khunti is a general practitioner in Leicester, a Senior Lecturer in the Department of General Practice and Primary Health Care, University of Leicester and a member of the National Diabetes Guideline development group.

Rhian Loudon is a general practitioner in Wolverhampton and a Lecturer in the Department of Primary Care and General Practice, University of Birmingham. She is sponsored by a National NHS R&D Primary Care Researcher Development Award.

Nicola Low has worked in sexual health and genito-urinary medicine for several years in London and Bristol. She is currently a Senior Lecturer in Epidemiology and Public Health Medicine in the Department of Social Medicine at the University of Bristol.

Bernadette Modell has worked for many years on risk identification and management of common inherited disorders, using haemoglobin disorders as a model. She is Emeritus Professor of Community Genetics at Royal Free and University College London Medical School, in the Department of Primary Care and Population Sciences and the Centre for Health Informatics and Multiprofessional Education.

Sangeeta Patel is a general practitioner in Balham, South London and a Lecturer in the Department of General Practice at St George's Hospital Medical School. She is sponsored by a National NHS R&D Primary Care Researcher Development Award.

Greta Rait is a general practitioner and MRC research fellow in the

Department of Primary Care and Population Sciences at the Royal Free and University College Medical School.

Aziz Sheikh is a general practitioner in West London, Chairman of the Research Committee of the Muslim Council of Britain and Senior Lecturer (PPP Post-Doctoral Fellow) at the Primary Care Epidemiology Unit, St George's Hospital Medical School, London.

Terminology used in this book

Available information about ethnic groups has often grouped different communities together unsatisfactorily. The more diverse ethnic categories used in the most recent 2001 census may facilitate more accurate and acceptable presentation of information in the future. Terms used in this book mean the following unless otherwise defined.

Black and minority ethnic group (BMEG)   There is no single unproblematic term that embraces all members of minority groups or that is completely acceptable to everyone. There is of course considerable heterogeneity between and within ethnic groups. There are many people from minority ethnic communities who do not identify themselves as 'black' but who, because of ethnic origin, language, cultural or religious differences, share a common experience of inequality, discrimination or racism. The use of 'black' and 'minority ethnic' together is intended to embrace those who may have this experience. However, it is recognized that the term is a compromise.

Ethnic group   A social group with a common sense of identity, as seen by both themselves and others, based on features such as language, religion, country of origin or customs.

Ethnicity   The social concept of ethnic identity, which may be self-defined or imposed by categorization by others. People identify themselves as belonging to a social grouping because they differ culturally in ways such as language, food, religions, lifestyle or geographical origin. Although group allegiance is dependent on culture it may also encompass physical features as in 'race' (see below). The perspective in this volume is that use of 'ethnicity' and an emphasis on culture is preferable to the term 'race', but it is recognized that others may use 'ethnicity' and 'race' synonymously.

'Race'   A biological concept referring to a group of people with a common inheritance and physical characteristic such as skin colour or facial features.

African-Caribbean   People of African descent from the Caribbean. Unless 'African' is defined separately, this term may also include people whose ancestry is in the African continent.

South Asian   This refers to a heterogeneous group of ethnic minority populations whose ancestral origins lie in the Indian subcontinent, that is, India, Pakistan, Bangladesh and Sri Lanka.

White   A term used to refer to those with European ancestral origins, describing the ethnic majority group of the UK. This is of course a heterogeneous group of people with diverse cultural backgrounds. Unless otherwise specified this may include white minorities such as the Irish and Traveller Communities.

Introduction

Joe Kai

We live in an ethnically diverse society. Yet the response from health services can be less than ideal. This book aims to provide a concise introduction to ethnicity and health care for health professionals, medical students and others in training. It seeks to be accessible and practical, rather than overly academic. Thus we hope it will assist busy practitioners and students to learn about and grasp the essentials necessary to respond effectively to ethnic diversity in health care.

The book focuses on primary care, where the majority of contact with health services take place. It is mainly intended for GPs, GP registrars, practice and community nurses, and other primary care team members, in addition to bilingual link workers, advocates and workers in social care. However, the general principles underlined in this volume are applicable to most health care settings. I therefore hope the book will be of interest and relevance to others, including professions allied to medicine.

Focus of the book

The book eschews 'multi-cultural' coverage of different ethnic groups, religions, beliefs, customs and practices. Sources of this information already exist for practitioners to acquire knowledge of relevance to local communities. However, a 'compendium' approach is problematic given the immensity of ethnic diversity, and may easily promote stereotyping.

Rather, this book emphasizes the need for health practitioners to:

♦   respond to individuals and recognize their diversity
♦   develop a broad understanding of the contexts and needs of communities
♦   adopt a generic approach using principles for good practice – for example, facilitating access to care, achieving effective communication, or developing sensitivity to stereotyping, prejudice and racism.

In many, if not most, respects the challenges for enhancing the health and health care of people from 'minority ethnic' communities are those common for all, in particular socially disadvantaged communities. Having underlined general principles for improving health care, the book then considers selected clinical topics and groups.

Content of the book

Ethnic diversity in context

This first section places the health of ethnically diverse communities in social and epidemiological context. Chapter 1 introduces the concepts of 'race', ethnicity and culture. It outlines the socio-economic, linguistic and religious features of diverse communities in the UK, highlighting experience of disadvantage and racism. Chapter 2 provides an overview of disease patterns among black and minority ethnic groups (BMEGs), noting the need to be careful in the interpretation and use of epidemiological information. It emphasizes that although there are ethnic differences in disease, the major health problems and priorities of BMEGs are similar to those of the majority population. Chapter 3 summarizes important general ways of improving quality of health care in a diverse society as a prelude to the next section.

Developing effective health care

This section contains seven chapters, each of which expands upon an essential facet of effective health care in more detail. Chapter 4 explains the vital importance of patient profiling to capture information on ethnicity, and how this can be achieved. Chapter 5 discusses aspects of access to health care, including how perpetuation of disadvantage may be subtle. It notes that 'ethnicity' is just one aspect of a person's identity that may interact with the characteristics of a service or health professional to influence access to care.

Chapter 6 considers how to achieve effective cross-cultural communication in health encounters. Chapter 7 describes models for interpreting and translation, and their operation. Chapter 8 explains the roles of bilingual link workers and advocates. It discusses ways of working with advocates and the challenges posed for both health practitioner and advocate. Chapter 9 outlines principles for effective health promotion and screening in ethnically diverse contexts. It emphasizes the need for community participation and describes the 'community educator' model by way of illustration.

Learning to respond diversity means more than achieving effective communication and overcoming language barriers. Chapter 10 focuses on other aspects of a generic approach important to any health encounter. Firstly, learning to value cultural diversity and responding to the individual. Secondly, becoming sensitized to our attitudes to difference – understanding stereotyping, prejudice and racism – and challenging their influence through our behaviour and the standards we set for practice.

Clinical care in practice

The third section of the book covers a range of clinical topics, health issues and groups that are arguably of particular concern for minority ethnic health in the

UK at the moment. This has meant difficult decisions about what to include in a deliberately slim volume. The 10 chapters in this section do not attempt to be comprehensive on their topic but cover essential points and practical guidance, pointing to a further bibliography where appropriate. These chapters include consideration of coronary heart disease (Chapter 11), diabetes (Chapter 12), hypertension and stroke (Chapter 13), mental health (Chapter 14), older people (Chapter 15), children and young families (Chapter 16), sexual health (Chapter 17), cancer and palliative care (Chapter 18), haemoglobin disorders (Chapter 19), and the health and care of refugees and asylum seekers (Chapter 20).

References provided at the end of chapters are not intended to be exhaustive. They contain selected publications, suggestions for further reading and other sources of further information where relevant.

Conclusion

Diversity can sometimes engender discomfort and uncertainty. It makes working in health care challenging but ultimately more vital and stimulating. Learning about ethnicity and health offers insights into how people from all walks of life may come to experience inequality. Crucially, learning to respond effectively to ethnic diversity can help health practitioners develop principles and an approach that they can apply to all people of whatever background, to the benefit of their patients and themselves. That is one value, among many, of valuing diversity.

Section I
Ethnic diversity in context

1 Ethnic diversity in social context

Mark R. D. Johnson

This chapter seeks to place black and minority ethnic groups (BMEGs) in the UK in social context. The concepts of ethnicity, race and culture are introduced. The challenges of describing the diversity of individuals and ethnic group are considered. The socio-economic experience, linguistic and religious features of diverse communities are then outlined, highlighting experience of disadvantage and racism.

Concepts of 'race', culture and ethnicity

The fallacy of 'race'

Trying to divide the population of the world into 'ethnic groups' is fraught with difficulty. Traditional anthropology defined four major human 'races', usually described as 'Caucasian' (white or European), 'Negroid' (Black or African), 'Mongoloid' (Asian, Chinese or Indic), and 'Australoid' (that is, the group of people described as 'Aboriginal' to Australia). These groupings arose from the idea of race as a bio-scientific concept assuming significant biological differences between populations. This concept of race is now firmly discredited by modern genetics. Over 99% of the genetic make-up of human beings is common to all ethnic groups.

Those differences that do exist between people and populations are minor and largely reflect superficial physical characteristics ('phenotypes') such as facial features, hair or skin colour. These differences remain the main way in which societies create artificial groups that are regarded differently and thus experience 'racial' discrimination. Thus the division of people into 'races' reflects social decisions rather than having any real scientific justification.

Culture and ethnicity

Culture is a complex social phenomenon and its definition problematic. It consists of the shared beliefs, values and attitudes that guide the behaviour of group members. Many people assume that culture is relatively static, but at the same time, assume that people can 'easily' change learned habits, 'if they want to'.

Table 1.1 Race, culture and ethnicity

Concept	Primary characteristics	Origin	Associated perceptions
'Race'	Inherent, biological, physical	Genetic – descent	Permanent
Culture	Behavioural expression of preferred lifestyle	Upbringing – learned	Capable of being changed, optional
Ethnicity or ethnic group	Identity, multi-faceted, 'political'	Socially constructed – internal or external or legal	Situational, negotiated

This ignores the value placed on personal history and the search for a stable, rooted identity. Recognizing and valuing cultural diversity in health encounters is considered in Chapter 10.

The concept of 'ethnicity' is more complex, but recognizes that people identify themselves with a social grouping on cultural grounds including, for example, language, lifestyle, religion, food and origins. The basis of 'ethnicity' is thus often a tradition of common descent and shared culture or history. It is essential to recognize that in a world of migration and mixing, cultures and societies are dynamic rather than fixed. Table 1.1 compares the concepts of race, culture and ethnicity.

The challenge of capturing diversity

When considering the causes of ill health and approaches to its prevention or care, it is necessary to consider the individual at risk, or the group to which they belong, in a holistic manner. The problem is using categories that most effectively describe factors relevant to, for example, susceptibility to poor health or health outcomes. It is difficult to manage without stereotypes and shorthand terms, but by using them we risk over-simplification and inappropriate generalization. How can we best describe people to capture diversity? Which aspects of this multidimensional concept are most important for the health practitioner?

Defining 'ethnic group'

The UK Race Relations Act 1976 defined a 'racial group' as 'a group of persons defined by reference to colour, race, nationality or ethnic or national origins ...' 'Ethnicity' and 'ethnic group' became more formally defined in UK law by a House of Lords decision (*Mandla* vs *Lee* 1983) as relating to those with 'a long shared history and a distinct culture'. Other 'relevant' characteristics were 'a common geographic origin or descent from a small number of common ancestors; a common language; a common literature; a common religion and being a minority within a larger community'.

For practical purposes, there is little alternative to using a selection of labels and categories. The ethnic groups identified by the Office of National Statistics in the decennial UK Census are usually adopted. Table 1.2 gives the ethnic categories that were used in the 1991 Census and those recently asked in the 2001 Census. Although the 2001 Census uses the term 'ethnic group', it also makes clear that this is seen as a matter of 'cultural background'.

Looking at Table 1.2, the reader might pause to consider to which ethnic group they would say they belong. Labelling one's own identity and 'ethnicity' can be seen to be difficult and inevitably subjective.

Table 1.2 Categories of ethnic group recorded in the UK Censuses of 1991 and 2001

1991	2001
White	White – British White – Irish White – Any other White background (please write in)
(Other . . .)	Mixed – White/Black Caribbean Mixed – White/Black African Mixed – White/Asian Any other mixed background (please write in)
Black – Caribbean	Black or Black British: Caribbean
Black – African	Black or Black British: African
Black – Other (please describe)	Black or Black British: Any other background (please write in)
Indian	Asian or Asian British Indian
Pakistani	Asian or Asian British Pakistani
Bangladeshi	Asian or Asian British Bangladeshi
Asian – Other (please describe)	Asian or Asian British Any other background (please write in)
Chinese	Chinese or Other Ethnic group Chinese
Any Other Ethnic Group (please describe)	Chinese or Other Ethnic group Any other (please write in)

Adapted from Office for National Statistics (ONS) forms. Reproduced with permission, Crown Copyright acknowledged.

The most recent Census questions reflect changes such as a tendency for some people of African-Caribbean origins born in Britain to determine their own identity as 'Black British'. The 2001 Census also asked people about their religion, which may make it easier to make projections of the numbers of people from the main religious groups, and anticipate the needs they may bring to the health service for religious observance, diet and counselling.

It is possible for new groups such as recent Kurdish or Bosnian refugees to be specifically coded by the 2001 Census under 'any other group', but there are no reliable statistics available on the numbers and locations of refugees and asylum seekers. They may not have completed the Census forms through fear of bureaucracy, many have been 'relocated' since arrival, and others will have come to Britain after 2001 (see Chapter 20).

Identifying ethnicity for research

For epidemiological research the tendency has been to rely on the commonly recorded variable 'country of birth', normally available on death certificates. However, at the time of the 1991 Census, over half the population in the 'Black' categories (54% Black Caribbean, 84% Black Other, and 36% Black African) were born in the UK, as were half of those giving their ethnic group as 'Pakistani', 42% of 'Indians' and 37% of 'Bangladeshis'. It is now estimated that less than 40% of the black and minority ethnic population can be identified by birthplace, and increasingly few by the birthplace of their parents. The problems of using 'country of birth' in examining variations in health are further discussed in the next chapter.

Summarizing components of ethnicity

Figure 1.1 demonstrates how some of the essential components of an ethnic group 'fit together'. All of these factors could affect the health needs of an individual. Using the right terms or questions can be very important in finding out about these issues. Aspects of 'culture', for example, may clearly be relevant to health and health care or promotion because of diet, attitudes toward tobacco or alcohol, or exercise. Language is clearly important to communication, and genetic background cannot be ignored as a 'risk factor' for certain conditions. Nationality may sometimes be relevant, for example reflecting refugee status, and the impact of the process of seeking asylum on mental or physical health.

The use of 'ethnicity', with its socially determined emphasis on culture, is preferable to 'race'. However the two are often used synonymously. Although the old term 'race' can no longer be used in scientific terms, it is often used in ordinary language as a shorthand term – implying 'those who are different from me'. Everyone has a 'race' or an ethnicity. Thus the use of the term 'ethnic' to mean 'people who are different from me' is both inappropriate and nonsensical.

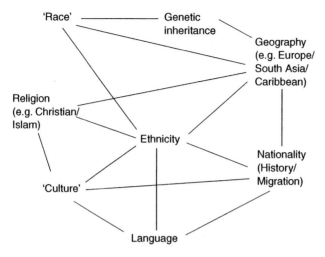

Figure 1.1 Components of 'ethnic group' and ethnicity

Ethnic diversity in Britain

Much of what we know about the geography and socio-economic profile of the black and minority ethnic (BME) population is based on the 1991 Census and will soon be superseded by the data from the 2001 Census. Some recent estimates on the size and nature of the BME population can be obtained from the 2000 Labour Force Survey (still using 1991 Census group categories). This suggests there are just over 4 million people living in Britain who consider they are from a minority ethnic group. This represents 7.1% of the UK population (see Figure 1.2).

Geographical distribution

The majority of people of BME origins live in the Greater London area or the Midlands, with smaller numbers in West Yorkshire and Greater Manchester, and other major metropolitan centres such as Liverpool and Cardiff. Relatively few live in rural areas.

Some towns or metropolitan boroughs become known for local concentrations of people from particular ethnic origins. For example, relatively large numbers of people from Somali backgrounds live in Liverpool, Sheffield, Cardiff and Birmingham. More than half the UK population of Bangladeshi origin lives in the East End of London, mostly in Tower Hamlets. The Vietnamese population, many of whom had been refugees in the 1960s and 1970s, have mostly moved to live in London, with smaller numbers in cities such as Nottingham and Derby. Similarly, Leicester has become known as a town whose economy has grown since the resettlement of Asian people (many

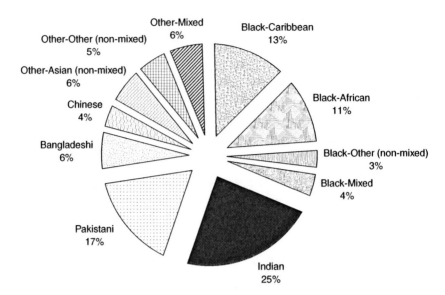

Figure 1.2 Distribution of total minority ethnic population by ethnic group. From Scott *et al.*[1]

Source: Scott A, *et al*. Sizes and chracteristics of minority ethnic populations of Great Britain – latest estimates. *Population Trends* 2001; 6–15.

of them Gujerati speakers) seeking asylum from events in East Africa in the 1970s, whereas Coventry's Asian population is predominantly Punjabi-speaking.

Birmingham has large populations of Punjabi, Pakistani (and/or Kashmiri) background, as well as a significant population of Caribbean background. The largest number of people of West African background are found in south-east London. The majority of people of South Asian origin in the northern towns of Yorkshire and Lancashire are of Pakistani origin, many of their forebears having moved from the Mirpur area of Kashmir. All of these, however, are generalizations.

Until the start of the dispersal programme run by the Home Office in 2000, most asylum seekers and refugees were likely to settle in London, unless they had relatives eleswhere or had been 'dispersed' in one of the earlier programmes for Polish, Ugandan Asian, Vietnamese or Yugoslav people. New areas of 'resettlement' currently include Birmingham, Glasgow, Liverpool, Leicester and Newcastle on Tyne (see Chapter 20).

Demography

The current demography of most BME populations is significantly different from that of the white majority. In particular, they tend to be younger, and with more children. This implies that one focus for health services should be on the needs of children, mothers and younger people, and health promotion to reduce disease in later life. At the same time the older minority ethnic population will increase very considerably over coming decades, with consequent implications for services and disease prevalence.

Total population fertility (the numbers of children in a family) has historically been greater, although this is now changing to resemble more closely the UK average. Among newer migrants (including most refugee populations) the sex ratio has been heavily skewed, so that men outnumber women, but this is no longer true for established populations.

Language

There is a constantly changing picture with the migration of new groups, including refugees, and the learning of English by settlers. Best current estimates are that there are more than 3 million speakers of other languages in England and Wales, but probably only 1% of these (300 000) have no ability in English. The remainder may, however, only have a very basic understanding of spoken English.

Recent estimates suggest over 300 languages are used as 'mother tongues' in London. Speaking a language does not, however, always imply literacy in that language, nor lack of English. Levels of skills in English also vary, both between people speaking different languages, and also from town to town between people who appear to be of similar ethnic origin. On current data, and over-generalizing, South Asian minority ethnic women – especially in Muslim cultural groups – are the least likely to speak or read English. They may also not be literate in their mother tongue.

Some languages, notably the Sylheti dialect of Bangladesh, do not have an agreed written form. Those who can speak Punjabi or a dialect variety of it, including Kashmiri forms such as Pahari and Mirpuri, may not be able to read it, or may read in Urdu or the 'Gurmukhi' (Devanagari) script. Many refugees and asylum seekers have very high levels of education, but their children's education will have been interrupted.

Religion

Numbers of Muslims in Britain are estimated variously at 1 million and 2 million. Less than 5% of 'Asian' groups say they have 'no religion', compared to about a third of the white population.[2] About half of the 'Indian' group interviewed in a national survey said they were Sikhs, and a further third were Hindu.[2] Religion is clearly very important to many people from a minority background, and may be a key part of their ethnic identity.

Care must be taken not to assume that ethnic groups are religious labels. It should be remembered, for example, that there are Christians of Pakistani, Bangladeshi and Indian origin. Many Vietnamese are members of the Roman Catholic faith, but others are Buddhist (as are many Indians and Chinese, and some Pakistanis).

Many evangelical Protestant churches have strong associations with African or Caribbean congregations. These are particularly popular among some younger people, whereas many of the older generation are members of the historic churches such as the Church of England, Presbyterian and Methodist, and the Roman Catholic tradition.

Socio-economic status and disadvantage

Historically, people from black and minority ethnic groups (BMEGs) have lived in areas of deprivation and have jobs of lower socio-economic status. This is often because of a history of exclusion and racial discrimination. Many 'ethnic differentials' in health status may be related as much to such deprivation as to ethnicity. There remain considerable differences in health between minority ethnic groups, which may be due to their varied experiences (in terms of geography, economy and migration history). However, 'ethnicity' remains important as a marker of need as well as a feature of individual identity.

Housing

About 19% of the white population live in areas described as 'council estates and low income areas', but about 40% of the Black and Indian groups, and as many as 63% of the Bangladeshi and Pakistani population live in such areas.[3] On the other hand, nearly a third (31%) of the white population live in areas described as 'affluent suburb, affluent family, or rural', compared to only 6% of those from Black, Pakistani or Bangladeshi backgrounds, and 14% of those with an Indian origin.

Other standard measures of deprivation, such as car ownership and housing tenure, are more problematic to analyse and interpret. Nearly two-thirds of Bangladeshi households have no car, compared to a third of white homes (in 1991). Indian households (1/4 with no car) appear to be better off.

Similarly, whereas two thirds of white families are in owner-occupied housing, this is true of only 40% of black African-Caribbean and one in three Bangladeshi households where social rented housing predominates. Nevertheless, overall four-fifths of South Asian households are owner-occupiers. Home ownership does not necessarily equate to affluence: in general, the prevalence of double glazing, garages, central heating and other such amenities are lower for South Asian home owners.

Employment

Black Caribbean or African, Bangladeshi and Pakistani men, are much more likely than whites to be employed in semi- or unskilled manual occupations. In contrast, Indian men are more likely to be of 'professional or managerial' status (13% compared to 8% of whites).

For the past 20 years, ethnic minority unemployment rates have been consistently double those of their white peers – and those for young people are double the rates of those aged between 25 and 50. Were higher numbers of South Asian (particularly Muslim) women to enter the employment market, these rates might worsen. Most of these women are probably acting as unpaid carers within their family and community networks.

These rates do not reflect 'unemployability' in terms of qualifications: ethnic minority youth are very similar to white youth in their levels of qualification, and more likely to continue education after school age. For example, in recent research Black Caribbean-origin men aged 20–24 were more than two and a half times as likely than whites to be in full-time post-compulsory education. African-Caribbean and Indian women were rather better qualified than their white peers.

Yet the industrial and occupational sectors in which ethnic minority employees are most likely to be found remain the less desirable, more insecure, or worst paid. Many ethnic minority employees thus work unsocial hours, shifts or longer hours, in order to maintain their incomes. In particular, ethnic minorities are still disproportionately employed in 'service', retail and transport occupations. Within such professions as medicine and nursing, those from minority ethnic backgrounds fill less popular specialities and shifts.

Racism

A convincing argument can be made that racism is hazardous to the health of BMEGs (Semmes 1996). There are some obvious ways in which this can happen. Racial attacks have become common events and a number of widely reported deaths such as that of Stephen Lawrence in 1993 have led to political action and considerable fear among communities.

Racial discrimination in housing and employment has led to many BME groups living in less good environmental settings, enjoying poorer working conditions and lower incomes and worse housing. Other forms of indirect or 'institutional' racism include issues such as lack of information in relevant languages, or appropriate to the diet, religion and culture of BMEGs; failure to plan services that are appropriate or accessible to BMEGs, and lack of training provided to health care staff. In particular, there is commonly a failure to monitor the use made of services to ensure that all groups have equitable access, according to their needs.

Fear of racial harassment may lead to avoidance of facilities such as parks, or a reduction in walking and taking exercise. Older people may avoid day centres, and mothers may be less likely to attend practices and antenatal clinics particularly at certain times. Fear of discrimination and the experience of verbal abuse (and seeing graffiti) can lead not only to mental distress, but possibly also to raised blood pressure and risk of physical disease. This, like the link between unemployment and ill health, has been contested, but there is no simple way of testing the hypothesis in a scientific study. Stress is known to have adverse health effects, and a climate of racism, xenophobia, or intolerance, might be reasonably assumed to cause stress.

The nature of racism and how health practitioners can respond is further discussed in Chapter 10.

Conclusion

There are many ways of describing people as members of 'ethnic' groups. These descriptions have effects and consequences for health care. It is important to consider both how a person thinks about or describes herself and himself, and how society treats people as 'ethnic groups'. Information on culture, religion and origins, and their careful consideration, are crucial to planning and providing health care. To ignore diversity is neither 'scientific' nor 'moral'. Indeed, it may risk causing further discrimination, exclusion and health inequality.

Key points

- Ethnicity is a complex concept comprising a number of dimensions of difference or diversity which should be taken into account in provision of health care
- The history of migration means that BMEGs tend to be concentrated in certain places but an 'ethnic group' label may conceal differences between groups of apparently similar origins living in different areas
- People within BMEGs may vary in their socio-economic status, religion, and language as well as in cultural practices
- Most BMEGs experience racism – direct, personal, indirect or institutional – which may affect their patterns of settlement as well as their socio-economic status and health
- Beware of making stereotypes from 'ethnic' labels

References

1. Scott A *et al.* Sizes and characteristics of minority ethnic populations of Great Britain – latest estimates. *Population Trends* 2001; 6–15.
2. Modood T, Berthoud R, Lakey J, Nazroo J, Smith P, Virdee S, Beishon S. *Ethnic minorities in Britain: diversity and disadvantage.* PSI Report 843, London: Policy Studies Institute, 1997.
3. *English Housing Survey.* London: DETR, 1998.

Further information

Acheson Report. *Independent inquiry into inequalities in health* (Chair: Sir Donald Acheson) London: Stationery Office, 1998.

Bhopal R. Is research into ethnicity and health racist, unsound, or important science? *BMJ* 1997; 314: 1751–1756.

Culley L, Dyson S (eds). *Ethnicity and nursing practice.* Basingstoke: Palgrave, 2001.

Evandrou M. Ethnic inequalities in health in later life. *Health Statistics Quarterly* 2000; 8: 20–28.

Johnson MRD, Owen D, Blackburn C, Rehman H, Nazroo J. *Black and minority ethnic groups in England: the second health and lifestyles survey.* London: Health Education Authority, 2000.

Nazroo JY. *The health of Britain's ethnic minorities.* London: Policy Studies Institute, 1997.

Semmes CE. *Racism, health and post-industrialism: a theory of African–American health.* Westport, CT: Praeger, 1996.

Much useful information is available online, including:

Health Survey for England: The Health of Minority Ethnic Groups '99 (Department of Health – *http://www.doh.gov.uk/public/england.htm*)

Ethnic Health in London: *http://www.doh.gov.uk/london/ethnic.htm*

London Health Observatory: *http://www.lho.org.uk/hil/bme.htm*

Health Care Needs assessment: *http://hcna.radcliffe-online.com/chapters.html*

2 Ethnic diversity in health and disease

Joe Kai and Raj Bhopal

Everyone tends to be curious about differences between people, both as individuals and as members of groups. Seeking to explain patterns of disease in populations, epidemiologists are drawn to the study of ethnic variations in health because this may generate hypotheses on why disease differences occur and help understand the causes of disease. The answers of course may benefit all populations. Famously, clues to the causes of heart disease were found by studying the mortality of Japanese Americans. They previously had very low rates of death from this cause, but these rose as they adopted an 'American' way of life.

Patterns of health and disease are profoundly influenced by socio-economic, environmental, genetic and cultural factors. This chapter concentrates on providing an epidemiological overview of disease patterns among black and minority ethnic groups (BMEGs) in the UK. The need to be careful in the interpretation and use of epidemiological information is highlighted.

There are significant ethnic differences in patterns of disease, both morbidity and mortality. However, the major health problems of ethnic minority communities, and therefore priorities for health improvement and health care, are similar to those of the majority population (e.g. cardiovascular disease and cancers). Much of the health inequality experienced by some minority ethnic groups may not result from their 'racial' and cultural background, but relate to their socio-economic disadvantage.

Information on ethnicity

The concepts of 'race' and ethnicity and the challenges of defining a person's ethnicity are discussed in the preceding chapter. Although there has been a statutory requirement for NHS hospitals to record the ethnicity of all 'admitted' patients since 1996, the collection, quality and use of such data remains variable. Thus reliable national statistics on hospital utilization by ethnic group are not available and information on patterns of morbidity is difficult to obtain. Ethnicity profiling of patients, and the particular importance of developing this in primary care where most formal health care interactions take place, is the subject of Chapter 4.

Using pragmatic ethnic group categories can fail to recognize important heterogeneity within a group. For example, 'South Asian' or 'Asian' is commonly used as a label for people born in, or descendants of those born in, India, Pakistan, Bangladesh and Sri Lanka. Yet Bangladeshi men have an extremely high prevalence of current smoking (49%) compared to all South Asian men (26%). Differing religious affiliations, for example Muslim, Hindu, Sikh, or Christian within this grouping may also impact on health.

The validity of health statistics for minority ethnic groups is based on several assumptions, for example that ethnicity categories are not only valid but consistently defined and ascertained; and that such designations are understood by the populations questioned. Currently, published information is most readily available for African-Caribbean and South Asian groups, is less in quantity and quality for people of Chinese origin, and virtually unavailable for most other groups, for example those from the Middle East and many groups of refugees. Sources of further guidance on the interpretation of epidemiological data and priorities are provided at the end of this chapter.[1]

Comparative and absolute perspectives

A traditional approach has been to compare the health of ethnic minority groups to that of the ethnic majority, that is, in Britain, the white population. This comparative perspective can be misleading when assessing health needs and service priorities. Consider Table 2.1 which shows disease patterns in males of Indian ethnicity and in men from the general population of England and Wales.

Comparing deaths using standardized mortality ratios (SMR), the differences between groups are emphasized (right-hand column: by rank order of SMR). For example, liver cancer or tuberculosis stand out as much more common in Indians compared to white males. These diseases might figure large when we think about this group's health. Yet it can also be seen that these conditions in fact account for few deaths. Now, if one considers absolute number of deaths (left-hand column: by rank order of number of deaths), the major fatal diseases for the minority group are seen to be similar to those of the population as a whole (heart disease, cerebrovascular disease, respiratory diseases, and cancers). For example, ischaemic heart disease accounts for many deaths among Indians, and rates of death are similar to those for white males.

This principle applies more generally. Although there are differences between all ethnic groups, the major diseases of the majority population are also very important to minority ethnic groups. Some major problems – such as heart disease, hypertension, stroke and diabetes – are particular priorities for certain groups (see below).

Table 2.1 Deaths and standardized mortality ratios (SMRs) in male immigrants from the Indian sub-continent (aged 20 and over; total deaths = 4352)

By rank order of number of deaths				By rank order of SMR			
Cause	Number of deaths	% of total	SMR	Cause	Number of deaths	% of total	SMR
Ischaemic heart disease	1533	35.2	115	Homicide	21	0.5	341
Cerebrovascular disease	438	10.1	108	Liver and intrahepatic bile duct neoplasm	19	0.4	338
Bronchitis, emphysema and asthma	223	5.1	77	Tuberculosis	64	1.5	315
Neoplasm of the trachea, bronchus and lung	218	5.0	53	Diabetes mellitus	55	1.3	188
Other non-viral pneumonia	214	4.9	100	Neoplasm of buccal cavity and pharynx	28	0.6	178
Total	2626	60.3	-		187	4.3	178

SMRs (= observed deaths/expected deaths' ×100) enable mortality comparisons after taking into account different variables such as age, sex and sometimes class. Comparison is usually to the experience of the population of as a whole. Hence a group whose mortality from a condition was the same as the latter would have an SMR of 100, if worse then over 100; if better then under 100. In the table the SMRs for the immigrant group are compared with the SMR for the male population of England and Wales, which was by definition 100.

From Senior P, Bhopal RS. Ethnicity as a variable in epidemiological research. *BMJ* 1994; 309: 327–330, including data originally published by Marmot et al.[3] Reproduced with permission of BMJ Publications.

Variations in mortality and morbidity

There are several major limitations to currently available data based on country of birth and death rates. For example, 'country of birth' is sometimes not fully and accurately identified on death certificates. Moreover, using 'country of birth' means data focus on older immigrants rather than British-born ethnic minorities (at the 1991 Census about half of BMEGs in the UK were born in Britain). Thus 'country of birth' does not equate to 'ethnic group'.

Table 2.2 shows data on deaths from selected causes by country of birth, in the period 1989–1992.

Note the above caution regarding SMRs in the absence of absolute numbers of deaths. SMRs are adjusted for age but not for social class (see below). SMRs cannot be compared either across the sexes or ethnic groups as age distributions differ by sex and ethnic group. They can only be compared in relation to the standard (i.e. 100) for each sex for the reference population, here the total population of England and Wales including all resident white and resident minority ethnic groups. Table 2.2 hides important variations within groups.

Nevertheless, bearing in mind the problems of such data, the health of some ethnic minority groups appears generally worse than that of the population as a whole for some diseases, for example ischaemic heart, cerebrovascular and hypertensive diseases, and diabetes. For other problems, such as cancers and respiratory diseases, the experience of BMEGs appears generally similar to or slightly better than that of the whole population. However, see further consideration of such variations below.

Patterns of morbidity are also complex with variations between, and within ethnic groups. Recent evidence from a national survey[2] relies on self-reported health but is based on self-identified ethnic group rather than country of birth. In general, those of Caribbean and in particular those of Pakistani and Bangladeshi origin report higher levels of ill health. In contrast, people of Chinese and Indian ethnicity report levels of health similar to or better than the white population. Detailed data on ethnic variations in mortality, and morbidity (patterns of consultation in general practice for different problems) are presented and discussed elsewhere.[1,4]

Why are there ethnic variations in health?

Explanations for ethnic inequalities in health experience are likely to reflect many inter-related factors. The influences of migration, genetic factors, culture, racism, access to services, and socio-economic status are all undergoing investigation.

Migration, genetic factors and culture

On balance, it does not appear that the stress of migration or poor health in the country of origin are responsible. However, evidence does confirm that immigrant

Table 2.2 Standardized mortality ratio (SMR) for selected causes by country of birth for 20–74 year olds, 1989–1992

Country of birth		Ischaemic heart disease	Cerebrovascular disease	Hypertensive disease	Cancers	Diabetes	Respiratory diseases
West/South Africa[a]	Men	58	261	764	106	297	118
	Women	61	162	780	111	156	49
Caribbean[b]	Men	62	205	471	89	439	61
	Women	86	197	748	91	697	57
Pakistan	Men	148	149	101	48	418	70
	Women	111	159	203	55	425	105
Bangladesh	Men	151	281	71	83	670	94
	Women	91	151	96	64	109	73
India	Men	142	134	145	59	317	85
	Women	158	146	159	70	333	91
Chinese[c]	Men	44	129	160	96	85	59
	Women	43	135	116	88	126	53
All people resident in England and Wales	Men	100	100	100	100	100	100
	Women	100	100	100	100	100	100

Data adapted from Gill et al.[1]

[a] Gambia, Ghana, Sierra Leone, Nigeria, Botswana, Zimbabwe, Lesotho, Swaziland.

[b] Jamaica, Barbados, Trinidad and Tobago, Guyana, Belize, West Indies, other Caribbean Islands.

[c] Hong Kong, China, Taiwan.

workers have largely occupied lower-paid jobs in the inner cities, which over time would be expected to have an adverse effect on health. Genetic factors are clearly important in relation to some haemoglobin disorders (see below). They may also potentially be associated with some problems such as heart disease, stroke or diabetes, inevitably interacting with other risk factors common to all populations (see chapters in Section II).

Exploring whether 'culture' may influence health is highly problematic because of vast diversity within ethnic groups. This includes lifestyles, behaviours, attitudes, social networks and cultural similarities between ethnic groups. Moreover the nature of culture is dynamic and context-specific, and inevitably overlaps with social and economic status.

Socio-economic status

Many ethnic variations in health may be largely the result of differences in socio-economic status rather than ethnicity *per se*.[4] This emphasizes a need to collect socio-economic information alongside ethnicity data when considering ethnicity and health.

On arrival in Britain most migrants held unskilled jobs. As discussed in Chapter 1 this legacy has been passed to their children (though there are many exceptions) and ethnic minority communities have more than their share of unemployment and low paid work. Much of the health inequality experienced by some ethnic minority groups may relate to their socio-economic disadvantage. Put in this wider context, the health and health care of many patients from ethnic minorities generates needs shared by all socio-economically disadvantaged communities. Thus the challenges and solutions for health improvement are likely to be similar.

Discrimination

Experience of racial harassment or discrimination may harm health as a result of social disadvantage, and inhibiting access to appropriate health care (see Chapters 1, 3 and 5). Racism may also directly affect health. Although there is a need for more research in the health arena,[5] racism is recognized as a factor influencing employment, housing and education which all affect health. Evidence in the US suggests a possible association between experience of racial discrimination and hypertension.

Lifestyle

All aspects of lifestyle which are important for the general population are important for ethnic minorities including smoking, alcohol, exercise, diet in relation to chronic disease, and stress. These must not be overlooked when undertaking health promotion with ethnic minorities. In addition, one should be alert to the potential relevance for some individuals of other cultural issues. Examples include self-treatment with herbal and other remedies, and a strong sense of modesty among some women which may have a bearing on their health (e.g. vitamin D deficiency related to lack of exposure to sunshine), health promotion (e.g. participation in physical exercise) and health care (physical examination).

Patterns of disease in minority ethnic groups

In considering disease patterns, four principles deserve emphasis:

- Ethnic minority groups are heterogeneous in their health, and there is heterogeneity within ethnic groupings.
- Do not assume the health of ethnic minorities is always worse than that of the ethnic majority: this is at best simplistic and sometimes wrong.
- In assessing expected level of health, recognize multiple influences on health such as socio-economic status, in addition to cultural, genetic or environmental factors.
- *Beware of stereotyping.* It is helpful to be aware of disease patterns that may be more or less common in some people, for example when considering a diagnosis. Such patterns may alert us to potential explanations or issues that may be relevant to care of a patient. However, stereotyping occurs when we fail to respond to people as individuals and inappropriately assume these patterns apply.

Simplifications may easily mislead. Detailed discussion of patterns of disease, mortality, lifestyle and health behaviours among minority ethnic groups can be found elsewhere[1,4] (and see 'Further information'). The following summarizes current knowledge about patterns of disease in ethnic minority groups bearing in mind the limitations of relevant information.

As noted above, both serious and minor health problems of most ethnic minority communities are similar to those of the population as a whole. For example, coronary heart disease, stroke and cancer are the commonest cause of death, and accidents, poisonings, digestive disorders, respiratory infection and circulatory problems the main reasons for admission to hospital whichever community you consider.

There are some ethnic differences in disease pattern. Some major diseases are more common in some ethnic groups, and therefore a heightened priority for their health. At the same time it should be remembered that problems that might be relatively less common in minority ethnic groups, such as respiratory diseases and cancers, still remain important and should not be ignored. From a population perspective these may be worth more attention than uncommon or rare conditions that happen to be relatively more common than in the white population, for example liver cancer.

Coronary heart disease

Coronary heart disease (CHD) (discussed in Chapter 11) is moderately higher in South Asian groups than in the population as a whole, with increasing evidence that the poorest groups, of Pakistani and Bangladeshi origin, have the highest rates. The causes of the excess are incompletely understood but socio-economic factors, lack of exercise, obesity, diabetes and insulin resistance appear significant. The classic CHD risk factors (high blood pressure, lipids, smoking) remain important and arguably most amenable to change. CHD is still one of the foremost killers of other ethnic groups including African-Caribbean and Chinese even though the rates are lower than in the population as a whole.

Stroke

The incidence of stroke is highest in African-Caribbean populations, but also the rates are relatively high in the Chinese and South Asian groups. The major known associated risk factor is hypertension (see Chapter 13), which is extremely common in African-Caribbean groups. Compared to white populations, hypertension appears to be similar in those of Indian and Pakistani origin and less common in Bangladeshis. This ethnic variation in hypertension is commonly, and possibly prematurely, attributed to genetic factors. Other causes, including racism, are being investigated. Stroke is an extremely important cause of death in all other ethnic minority populations.

Cancer

Overall, cancers tend to be less common in ethnic minority groups than in the white comparison population (but a dominant problem, nonetheless). Some cancers are, comparatively speaking, strikingly less common, for example lung cancer – relating to lower smoking prevalence. Nevertheless, this cancer remains the top ranking cancer in men in most ethnic groups. Oropharyngeal cancers are more common in South Asian groups and prostate cancer is more common in African origin groups. Cancer variations are usually attributed to environmental factors. Cancer and palliative care are discussed in Chapter 18.

Diabetes

Diabetes (see Chapter 12) is much commoner in African-Caribbean and South Asian minority groups than in the population as a whole. Prevalence in the Chinese may be similar to the white population but, on the basis of a higher prevalence of impaired glucose intolerance in women, there is evidence that a rise is imminent. The causes of the high rates are likely to be a mix of genetic, lifestyle, environmental and economic factors.

Respiratory diseases

These diseases tend to get little attention. The mortality and morbidity from them, for example chronic obstructive pulmonary disease (COPD), is usually a little less than in the white comparison populations. This makes them very common and important problems which ought not to be neglected.

Infectious diseases

Infections such as common respiratory and gastrointestinal diseases are dominant and important in all ethnic groups. Diseases that are associated with warm climates such as malaria are much more likely in ethnic minority groups. Tuberculosis is commoner in most ethnic minority groups, particularly South Asian ones. The causes are complex – relating to opportunities for exposure (travel, migration, etc.), immunity and living conditions in the UK. The latter seems to be an important factor maintaining the high level of tuberculosis in South Asians settled in the UK.

Haemoglobinopathies

Haemoglobinopathies are the subject of Chapter 19. They include thalassaemias and sickle cell disorders, important genetic conditions that affect people who originate from Africa, the Caribbean, the Middle East, Asia and the Mediterranean.

Childhood mortality

Perinatal and neonatal mortality rates, and those in the age group 1–14, tend to be higher in most studies. The exception is the comparatively low incidence of sudden infant death syndrome demonstrated in some ethnic minority groups. The causes are complex and poorly understood. The high perinatal mortality rate among Pakistanis may be partly linked to consanguineous marriages, but this remains controversial. These marriages can lead to an increase in rare recessively inherited disorders, but the effect of this on the disease patterns of the population as a whole has been exaggerated. Chapter 19 discusses this issue further.

Mental health

Evidence here is limited, difficult to interpret, and controversial. As elsewhere, variations may reflect socio-economic factors rather than ethnicity. Differences in 'pathways into health care' for different ethnic groups (such as difference in the expression of illness, its detection and diagnosis, or the way illness is managed) may influence the patterns of mental ill health reported from hospital or treatment statistics. A further consideration is the reliability and cultural sensitivity of instruments, including clinical history taking, used to assess mental ill health in different ethnic groups. Health professionals' understanding and assumptions about the mind, body and disease may not be shared by patients with a different culture (see Chapter 14).

Compared to the general population, African-Caribbeans may have higher rates of depression and are more likely to be admitted to hospital with a diagnosis of schizophrenia; South Asian groups have about the same rate of psychosis and appear to have lower rates of anxiety and depression, though evidence on depression in particular is conflicting. Overall those born in the Caribbean and South Asia have lower rates of suicide, but young women born in India and East Africa have higher rates of suicide. Information about white minority communities is very limited but suggests lower rates of mental ill health among the Chinese and higher rates of anxiety, depression and psychosis among those of Irish origin. This summary oversimplifies a complex picture.[6]

Sexual health

A high prevalence of sexually transmitted disease including gonorrhoea and chlamydia has been reported among African-Caribbeans. The risk of HIV among pregnant women from sub-Saharan Africa is much higher than that of other populations, with little evidence of HIV in women born in Southern Asia or UK-born South Asian communities. Fertility in Pakistani and Bangladeshi women has been reported as more than double that of white women, and associated with lesser use of contraception. Individual aspirations and attitudes to family may vary. Enhancing communication and cultural sensitivity in provision of family planning services remain important in addressing potentially unmet needs. Sexual health is discussed further in Chapter 17.

Conclusion

When considering health and disease in ethnic groups it is important to recognize both similarities and differences between groups. There are ethnic differences in disease patterns but ethnic similarities in health priorities. Health services and practitioners face a challenge. They must ensure they prioritize the important and common causes of death and disability shared by all communities. However, they must also respond to more specific patterns of disease in their local population as an integral part of their approach. For many patients from ethnic minorities the issues for their health and health care are shared with other socio-economically disadvantaged communities.

Essential points

- Take care when interpreting epidemiological information concerning ethnicity
- The major diseases and health problems of most minority ethnic groups are similar to the population as a whole (e.g. coronary heart disease, stroke, cancer)
- There are some ethnic differences in disease patterns
- Beware of stereotyping
- Much ethnic variation in health may reflect socio-economic differences rather than ethnicity

Acknowledgements

Part of this chapter draws upon other work we have conducted with colleagues, in particular Sarah Wild and Paramjit Gill, whose contributions we gratefully acknowledge.

References

1. Gill PS, Kai J, Bhopal RS, Wild S. Health care needs assessment of black and minority ethnic groups. In: *NHS health needs assessment, the fourth series of epidemiologically based reviews.* Oxford: Radcliffe, 2003. Available online at *http://hcna.radcliffe-oxford.com/bmegframe.htm.* This discusses detailed data on ethnic variations in mortality and morbidity (patterns of consultation in general practice for different problems), lifestyle and health behaviours among minority ethnic groups, and provides guidance on the interpretation of epidemiological data and priorities.
2. Senior P, Bhopal RS. Ethnicity as a variable in epidemiological research. *BMJ* 1994; 309: 327–330.
3. Marmot MG, Adelstein AM, Bulusu L, Shukla V. *Immigrant mortality in England and wales 1970–78* (OPCS Studies on Population and Medical Subjects No.47). London: HMSO,1984.
4. Nazroo J. *The health of Britain's ethnic minorities. Findings from a national survey.* London: Policy Studies Institute, 1997.
5. Bhopal RS. Is research into ethnicity and health racist, unsound, or important science? *BMJ* 1997; 314: 1751–1755.
6. Nazroo J. *Ethnicity and mental health. Findings from a national community survey.* London: Policy Studies Institute, 1997.

Further information

Bhopal R. Ethnicity and race as epidemiological variables. In: Macbeth H, Shetty P (eds). *Health and ethnicity.* London: Taylor & Francis, 2001.
Department of Health. *Health survey for England.* London: HMSO, 1999. Available online at *http://www.doh.gov.uk*

3 Toward quality in health care for a diverse society

Joe Kai

> I was feeling sick, sick, and pains here. My doctors saying 'flu' and then
> 'stress'. I go to the Casualty and it was the heart attack and sugar too high...I
> no English. Doctors no Punjabi. My boy speaks to doctors for me. Now I am
> too tired. I have to go back to hospital but not understand what for...
> [Patient speaking through interpreter]

Our societies are increasingly diverse. However, as the account above suggests,
the response from health services is often found wanting. The experiences of
people from black and minority ethnic groups (BMEGs) provide a window into
understanding how people in society may come to suffer inequalities in health
care and health. Many challenges for improving care are common to all communities, particularly those who are socially disadvantaged. Thus what follows
should be regarded as a logical and integral part of improving health care for all.

Most people from BMEGs do not want different services from the majority
population. They just want good quality services – like everyone else.
Fundamentally, this means the ability to identify and respond to the differing
needs of individuals. This chapter summarizes important ways of enhancing
quality of health care for people from diverse communities, before their discussion in more detail in subsequent chapters. Although the focus is on primary
care, these principles apply to other health care settings.

Effective access to appropriate care

Most people from BMEGs have consultation rates with their GP that are higher
than or similar to those of the general population.[1] However, this does not mean
people from minority ethnic populations experience effective access to appropriate health care.

Higher GP consultations may reflect greater ill health and social disadvantage. They may also be due to many other factors. These include poorer communication within, or poorer outcomes from consultations, less well-developed
primary care in the inner city, and care insensitive to differing cultural needs or

based on stereotyping. There is also some evidence that access to specialist care, for example investigation and surgical treatment of cardiovascular disease, may be poorer for some people from BMEGs although this is contentious. All of these may compromise quality and outcomes of care, and potentially contribute to the inequalities in health described in Chapter 2.

Patients' perspectives

Effective communication with health practitioners is a dominant issue.[2] In common with the majority population, people from BMEGs underline the importance of being given time, being listened to, being examined and given appropriate explanation. Yet these basic requirements may commonly not be met. In particular they may experience negative attitudes and cultural insensitivity from professionals.[2,3] Language barriers and lack of availability of interpreting create major problems. Adding to these difficulties, people may feel uninformed about different services and how to access them. The preferences of some people for health professionals of similar ethnicity and gender to themselves are also unlikely to be met.

Health professionals providing primary care

In common with their patients, GPs may recognize the challenges of communication and understanding patients' culture. However, GPs often give most prominence to the realities of primary care in socially disadvantaged settings whatever the population: for example, problems of pressure on time and resources, high frequency of consultation about 'minor' illness, patients' multiple 'social' problems and high prevalence of psychological distress. Similarly, GPs draw attention to the difficulties of health promotion and care of chronic disease such as diabetes and heart disease, when people in deprived settings may have other priorities and stressors in their lives.

Time to get real about quality of care

There are compelling reasons to 'get real' about quality of care for a diverse society. People from BMEGs form a growing proportion of the general population (Chapter 1). They represent or will come to represent ethnic majorities in several of our cities. Increasing intra-urban and intra-regional migration of families, and the dispersal of refugees across the country (Chapter 20) mean there will be few places that do not enjoy ethnic diversity.

At the same time, epidemiological evidence shows experience of health inequality and the health needs of many people from BMEGs is considerable and rising. They have an already high prevalence of major disease and BMEGs will form an increasing proportion of older people (Chapters 1 and 2).

Although research is still needed, it is possible to recommend steps to enhance health care for people from BMEGs (see Box 3.1). Crucially these

---

Box 3.1   **Steps to improve quality of care**

Patient profiling

- Gathering and using ethnicity information

Removing barriers to access

- Empowering reception staff
- Raising awareness of services and health issues
- Improving physical accessibility and appointment systems
- Culturally acceptable provision

Enhancing effective communication

- Attending to general principles of good communication
- Negotiating language and cultural barriers with bilingual support

Learning to respond to diversity and difference

- Developing local cultural knowledge
- Responding to the individual
- Awareness of attitudes: stereotyping, prejudice, and racism

Appropriate health education and promotion

Developing a diverse workforce

Working with communities

Support to disadvantaged settings: tackling inequalities

Facilitating change

---

should form part of local plans for clinical governance, a new imperative for NHS organizations to be accountable for improving and safeguarding standards in order to provide high quality care.[4] Moreover their implementation will help the NHS meet its legal duty under the new Race Relations Amendment Act (2000). This requires all public authorities to not merely avoid discrimination but also take positive steps to promote race equality.

The remainder of this chapter summarizes these steps. Similar principles apply to all services. The reader should refer to chapters in Section II of this book for further detail. In particular, Chapter 5 discusses how identities of an individual patient, health professional and service characteristics may interact to determine ease of access.

Patient profiling

Profiling of patients, including data on their ethnicity, is a prerequisite for understanding and defining local populations, assessing needs, and subsequent development of services. Unfortunately the NHS does not gather this information consistently and appropriately.

Data should include self-defined ethnicity (usually by Census category – see Chapter 1), language, religion and other needs. Patients and professionals need to be aware of the purpose of data collection and supported by training to seek information sensitively and accurately. This information must then be used to improve quality of care through audit and evaluation. Patient profiling in primary care is the subject of Chapter 4.

Removing barriers to access

Empowering reception staff

Receptionists and other administrative staff are usually the first important point of contact with patients. They can play a pivotal role in facilitating access to services. Recruitment of staff to reflect the diversity of the local population can be an important starting point (see below). Practices and other services should ask if their reception staff are enabled through their service organization and training to, for example:

- facilitate telephone access for appointments
- promote access to relevant information about services
- liaise with bilingual services (e.g. identifying need and booking an interpreter)
- be sensitive to patients' gender preferences for health professional
- appropriately seek and record patient profiling and ethnicity information.

Raising awareness of services and health issues

Use by, and awareness among BMEGs of community services, such as community nurses, chiropody, dentists and opticians, and local authority services such as home care support and meals on wheels, appears to be lower than average. Although uptake of childhood immunizations is similar or higher than average, uptake of cervical screening and breast screening has been generally low. Services should consider:

- Do they have readily available signs, leaflets, audiovisual displays and resources that are accurate and appropriate to local communities in relevant languages?
- Have they identified, developed and used information to inform patients about health issues (e.g. health promotion, mental ill health, heart disease) and services (e.g. how to register with a dentist)?
- Are they collaborating with local community and voluntary organizations, press, radio, TV, and schools to raise awareness?

Physical accessibility and appointment systems

Examples of questions services might consider include:

◆ Is there appropriate flexibility, for example longer appointments where interpreting is required, surgeries that include open access options, the timing of surgeries and clinics?

◆ Are facilities secure and well lit? In a recent national survey 58% of people from minority ethnic groups avoid going out at night and 35% visit shops at certain times only because of concerns about racial harassment.[5]

Culturally sensitive care

Although services should be acceptable to all patients, they should be sensitive to the cultural values and beliefs of people from BMEGs and seek to offer appropriate choices in care. Staff learning to respond to diversity and difference is vital here (see below). Health services must ask questions of the care they provide. For example:

◆ Are health promotion and education programmes adapted to cultural and religious backgrounds and provided in appropriate media and languages?

◆ Do meals in community day centres, nursing homes or respite nursing care meet religious and dietary requirements?

◆ Are there quiet rooms or prayer space which are not dominated by symbols of the majority religion and suited to religious observance by other faiths?

◆ Are female health professionals available? Women from all minority ethnic groups (except the Chinese), in particular Pakistani and Bangladeshi women, appear more likely than white women to prefer to consult a female doctor, probably reflecting the cultural and religious traditions of Muslim groups.

Enhancing effective communication

The central importance of effective communication in health encounters is self-evident. Achieving this means addressing the following:

Attending to the general principles of good communication

Good communication with any individual involves the principles of showing courtesy, interest and respect, active listening and responding to non-verbal cues and so on. Unsurprisingly, these basic requirements are as important for people from BMEGs as anybody else. These and other aspects of cross-cultural communication are discussed in Chapter 6.

Negotiating language and cultural barriers with bilingual support

Language barriers are major obstacles to care, notably for women and older people from South Asian and Chinese populations, and those from refugee communities. Of those who have difficulty communicating with their GP, less than 10% may have access to a trained interpreter, and around 75% use a friend or relative to translate for them. A third of people may still feel their GP has not understood them.[5]

Recruitment of bilingual staff from BMEGs or learning elements of local languages is helpful. However, health professionals can most improve this dismal situation by working with professional trained interpreters, or using telephone-based interpreting. Of course, they must make their patients aware that such help is available. The benefits are obvious:

> She is a good GP and she listens carefully. She normally arranges an interpreter for me, and has referred me to a specialist when I need it. I would recommend my GP to all refugee women with children.[2]

Unfortunately trained interpreters tend to be underused. Professionals need to recognize that allowing friends or family to interpret for patients is usually unsatisfactory. They may also need to learn the skills to work effectively with trained interpreters. These issues are discussed further in Chapter 7.

Professionals can further enhance effective communication, understanding, and consultation outcomes by working with link workers and advocates. They can help negotiate cultural barriers and inequalities in power between professionals and patients (see Chapter 8).

Learning to respond to diversity and difference

Cultural sensitivity

Effective communication means more than overcoming language barriers. Professionals can acquire locally relevant cultural knowledge and understanding, for example, about beliefs, diet and religion (see 'Further information' below) in addition to patterns of disease presentation and management (see Section III). However, it should be remembered that 'cultural sensitivity' is often more about showing some respect and common sense then 'knowing' about someone's culture:

> The nurses...think my grandmother should wear a jogging suit instead of a sari to make it easier to dress and undress her. It's strange to even suggest that an old lady who has worn a sari all her life should wear jogging pants. Their (the community nurses') values are different to ours. The old lady is confused as it is...we don't think it right to rob her of her remaining dignity [Gujerati woman caring for a grandmother with dementia][6]

Responding to individuals and 'difference'

Clearly no 'knowledge based' training can prepare professionals for all the issues that ever increasing diversity creates. Learning generic skills to respond flexibly to all encounters is more appropriate. In other words, responding to each patient as an individual, with individual needs, and to variations in patients' culture in its broadest sense.

As with the majority population, professionals must acknowledge the cultural context in which health and illness is expressed. For example, any patient, black or white, will have a particular ethnicity, education, socio-economic background, or set of health beliefs and experiences.

Responding to this diversity demands a heightened awareness of our response to difference and our attitudes. This means developing sensitivity to, stereotyping, prejudice and racism – and how this can be challenged. These issues are considered further in Chapter 10.

Health education and promotion

Health education and promotion strategies often neglect the needs of people from BMEGs. For example a smaller proportion have given up smoking (e.g. Bangladeshi men) compared to the white majority. Practitioners and Primary Care Trusts should beware over-emphasis on cultural 'differences'. The health priorities of minority ethnic groups (e.g. CHD and social inequality) may be very similar to the majority population (see Chapter 2). Indeed health beliefs, attitudes and education needs of communities are often more similar than expected.

Targeting and delivering health promotion may require a different, flexible approach. Health professionals need to establish the community's views and aspirations; their reactions to proposed methods and settings; and the effects of interventions not only on the target health issue but also on the wider aspects of the community's life. Health promotion and screening for BMEGs forms the subject of Chapter 9, and relevant aspects in relation to different clinical areas are discussed in Section III.

Developing a diverse workforce

Over 7% of NHS staff are from BMEGs. Local health care workforces should reflect the ethnic diversity of local communities. This means shifts in organizational culture and recruitment. The new Race Relations Amendment Act may help (see above).

Discrimination may reduce the numbers of BME people seeking employment in health services. Black and Asian junior doctors are more likely than white ones to report workplace bullying. Services should have clear procedures for dealing with racism and racial harassment towards or from staff and patients. These policies need to be publicized to both staff and patients.

Many patients from BMEGs have countered their linguistic disadvantage by consulting GPs who are fluent in their own language. The imminent retirement of a cohort of these doctors from minority ethnic backgrounds who have sustained general practice in many disadvantaged areas is a cause for concern.

Potential to attract a younger generation of doctors, nurses and other health professionals who may share ethnicities and languages with their patients exists. However, such potential cultural competencies must not be assumed nor inappropriately exploited. In primary care opportunities such as salaried GP and nurse practitioner schemes with flexible options for professional development in teaching, research or clinical speciality need to be pursued.

Recruitment, in particular to nursing and professions allied to medicine, needs to be improved. Cultural or material constraints, lack of educational opportunities, and discrimination must be addressed. This is important. For example, some patients identify the lack of 'anyone like me' in a ward as a stressful factor affecting their recovery. Creative outreach approaches may help, for example by awareness raising in schools and colleges to encourage young people to apply for and enter health related and health professional access courses.

These approaches can be allied to partnerships with local communities that enable development of community members through accredited training to facilitate routes to higher education. Examples of such practice are emerging.[7]

Working with communities

Many issues for appropriate service provision (e.g. effective access to services or care of chronic disease) are likely to be shared with other communities of interest, in particular those from disadvantaged white populations.

Local communities and their expertise – organizations, voluntary groups, and individuals – should be valued and engaged wherever possible in the strategies suggested in this chapter. These may include community consultation about health needs or developing services (e.g. developing local interpreting services, health promotion interventions, ethnic recruitment to the workforce or approaches to patient profiling). A range of approaches can be used including community development and participatory research.[7]

Tackling inequalities: support to disadvantaged settings

Approaches to improving health need to be set within the wider context of social exclusion and inequality in which many people from BMEGs experience health. Thus they should be part of wider policy towards employment, housing and equality of opportunity including multi-agency responses to address racism.

Improving primary care for many patients from BMEGs will require targeting of resources and support to disadvantaged areas of most need. Examples include developing inadequate practice premises or addressing poor staff recruitment and high staff turnover by investing in more flexible career options (see above).

There are opportunities to move beyond traditional biomedical models of health service provision to their integration with more socially oriented and holistic approaches to health improvement. They include urban regeneration initiatives (Single Regeneration Budget), Health Action Zones, New Deal for Communities, Sure Start and the new flexibilities that may arise from integrating health and social services. The limited but emerging evidence on effective ways of reducing health variations must be capitalized upon.[8]

Facilitating change

A question of commitment

General awareness of ethnic diversity and health care remains low. It requires a higher profile politically and among health professionals, for example during their training. Commitment of resources driven by government with, hereto neglected, monitoring of the implementation of policy and its evaluation is needed (performance management).

Learning from experience

There is some indication about what is needed to enhance the quality of primary care for people from BMEGs but less guidance about how to do it. The dissemination of models of implementation and good practice is thus vital. Examples are outlined throughout subsequent chapters of this book.

Meanwhile, research into ethnicity and health has largely failed to improve health care for ethnic minorities. Greater use of patient ethnicity profiling and the potential evaluation of clinical governance will help. To facilitate change, the focus of research needs to shift from the repeated definition of similar problems (of access to care or disease risk for example) to research that provides evidence about the implementation and effectiveness of interventions to improve quality of care and health outcomes.

Key points

◆ Most people from diverse ethnic communities do not want 'different' services. Like everyone else they just desire good quality services (e.g. effective communication in health encounters)

- Identify and respond to the differing needs of individuals
- Consider and follow steps to improve quality of care (see Box 3.1 above)
- Many challenges for improving care are common to all, particularly socially disadvantaged communities

References

1. Gill PS, Kai J, Bhopal RS, Wild S. Health care needs assessment of black and minority ethnic groups. In: Raftery J, Mant J, Stevens A. (eds). *The epidemiologically based health needs assessment reviews. Third series.* Abingdon: Radcliffe, 2003. Available online at *http://hcna.radcliffe-oxford.com/bmegframe.htm.*
2. Fassil J. *Primary health care for black and minority ethnic people: a consumer perspective.* Leeds: NHS Ethnic Health Unit, 1996.
3. Yee L. *Breaking barriers: towards culturally competent general practice.* London: Royal College of General Practitioners, 1997.
4. Scally G, Donaldson L. Clinical governance and the drive for quality improvement in the new NHS. *BMJ* 1998; 317: 61–65.
5. Nazroo J. *The health of Britain's ethnic minorities.* London: Policy Studies Institute, 1997.
6. Katbamna S, Bhakta P, Ahmad W, *et al.* supporting South Asian carers and those they care for: role of the primary health care team. *British Journal of General Practice* 2002; 52: 300–305.
7. Kai J, Hedges C. Minority ethnic community participation in needs assessment and service development in primary care: perceptions of Pakistani and Bangladeshi people about psychological distress. *Health Expectations* 1999; 2: 7–20.
8. Arblaster L, Lambert M, Entwhistle V, *et al. Review of research on the effectiveness of health service interventions to reduce variations in health.* Report No.3, NHS Centre for Reviews and Dissemination: York University, 1996.

Further information

The Health Development Agency commissions and publishes relevant reports, research and other guidance concerning minority ethnic health, and other work of relevance to improving health and health care. These are free and can be downloaded from the HDA website (*http://www.hda-online.org.uk*). They include a useful compilation entitled *Health-related resources for black and minority groups (second edition).*

The King's Fund (*http://www.kingsfund.org.uk*) has a range of free downloadable reports and articles concerning minority ethnic health, in addition to relevant publications available from its bookshop.

Texts describing cultural aspects of different ethnic groups include:

Karmi G (ed.) *The ethnic health handbook: a fact file for health care professionals.* Oxford: Blackwell Science, 1996. This handbook provides cultural information on over twenty ethnic groups and five different religions, including, for example, coverage of naming systems and titles; religious festivals, obligations and practices; diet; social customs; and cultural issues concerning birth and death.

Sheikh A, Gatrad AR (eds). *Caring for Muslim Patients*. Abingdon: Radcliffe, 2000. This book seeks to promote better-informed dialogue about the interface between faith and health. It profiles the Islamic worldview and its concepts of health and disease. Muslim practices and customs of relevance to health and health care are explored and illustrated.

Helman C. *Culture, health and illness*, 4th edn. London: Arnold, 2001. This provides a perspective on medical anthropology applied in a clinical context.

Section II
Developing effective health care

4 Patient profiling in primary care

Ben Jones and Katy Gardner

Effective health needs assessment and appropriate service delivery requires a detailed understanding of the demography, morbidity and health care utilization of communities. Considerable variations exist in health, and in access to and use of health services, among groups defined by country of birth and ethnicity. Yet our ability to determine morbidity and health care use for black and minority ethnic (BME) populations, particularly in primary care, remains limited.

Few primary health care teams collect information about the ethnicity of their patients or use this information to inform decisions about health care provision. Providers of in-patient services in secondary care have been required to collect information about ethnicity of patients since 1995, yet information has not been collected systematically and has been little used.

Although 'ethnic monitoring' has also been advocated in primary care for some time it is only recently being adopted by some practices and Primary Care Trusts (PCTs). The information gained from a more accurate profile of the practice population can be used in a number of ways including:

- targeting service provision more closely to need
- identifying the individual needs of patients, including culturally appropriate care
- targeting 'at risk groups' for health promotion
- using the information to improve health outcomes
- informing resource allocation.

This chapter provides examples of how this can happen. It highlights the opportunities created to better understand what influences access to health care.

Patient profiling

Ethnicity profiling must be done systematically or not at all. It should be a routine and integral part of the wider information gathering necessary for institutions to provide appropriate and effective services for all patients, of whatever background or need (requirements of the 2000 Race Relations Amendment and

1995 Disability Discrimination Act). Thus the term 'patient profiling' is preferred to 'ethnic monitoring'.

Practices and local communities must be fully involved from the start. Patient profiling benefits the whole population, not just people from BME communities. Ultimately patient profiling (including ethnicity) should ideally become part of the GP registration process, and in the future be entered onto a smart card or electronic record to be available throughout the NHS. Above all, patient profiling is about using the data to make a difference.

Key issues and challenges

The main challenges in developing patient profiling in primary care are:

◆ gaining its acceptance by patients and staff
◆ implementing appropriate methods
◆ using the information
◆ funding and sustainability.

All these are possible and can be achieved. Introducing the process may meet with uncertainty, fear and a lack of knowledge. There may be little grasp of the importance of ethnicity or how primary care staff can make a difference. Ownership of the process is crucial, but staff may already feel swamped with other service and policy priorities such as National Service Frameworks. To get them to prioritize a currently voluntary process is hard. Communities too, who have much to gain, are those most likely to have suffered from 'survey fatigue' in the past, for no visible benefit.

The use of patient profiling data can also be hamstrung by a lack of epidemiological and data handling skills in primary care. The recent advent of PCTs in the NHS embracing public health functions and skills may lead to greater integration of these skills into primary care. Patient profiling should play an important role in the new NHS culture of information. It must provide high quality data that is a credit to the investment.

Finally, patient profiling cannot be done for nothing. The greater and welcome emphasis placed on reducing health inequalities and improving the health of BME communities in the 2000 NHS plan now needs to be accompanied by appropriate resource and performance management to support this vital development.

Patient profiling in practice

Putting patient profiling into practice is not difficult. Different areas have gone about it in different ways. What follows are the lessons we have learned from 4 years of work in Liverpool.

Key individuals with a reputation for championing change must be identified within and without the NHS. These might be directors of public health, local councillors or community leaders. They can help, for example, in deciding what information to seek from patients, to facilitating action based on the data collected.

What data should be sought?

The decision about what data to collect can be driven by local needs. In general they should consist of variables that are unlikely to change much over time. 'Self-identified ethnic group', 'country of birth', 'language read and spoken', and 'need for an interpreter' should form the basis of the dataset. Information about access needs for people with disabilities may be collected (e.g. need for loop system, large print, Braille). Additional data might also reflect local priorities or particular practice issues such as identifying carers, or the time spent waiting for appointments.

Patient profiling should primarily be considered as obtaining essential data for audit to improve quality of care, rather than as 'research' although it clearly might contribute to the latter. It is important the process is not too ambitious. There is a wide range of data that might appear interesting to collect but they should be limited to what can be used in practice: 'information is for action'. An example of a data collection form is shown in Figure 4.1. Further examples can be obtained from the useful contacts listed at the end of the chapter.

Involving community and staff

In Liverpool contacts were established with local community groups from the outset through existing networks, a local health forum, community newspapers and the mosque. Once the advantages of patient profiling had been explained and issues of confidentiality were clarified, communities were enthusiastic.

Staff training is essential, not only to involve staff but to give them the confidence to approach the subject of ethnicity with patients. All practice staff, including the clinical team, need to be involved. Training in Liverpool is in two parts.

◆ The first addresses cultural diversity and gives a background and local examples of varying morbidity and mortality between different ethnic groups. The training challenges perceptions about equality of access, ideas that all patients 'should be treated in the same manner' and why data that is already available is insufficient.

◆ The second part of training is a guide to the roles of staff in data collection. In our experience this has increased the commitment of staff to the process as well as equipping them to deal with patients' enquiries.

إذا احتاج للمساعدة في تعبئة هذه الاستمارة ، فضلا تحدث مع موظف قسم الاستقبال في عيادة طبيبك

ফর্মটি পূরন করতে সাহায্যের দরকার হলে আপনার
ডাক্তারের সার্জারির লিঙ্কপার্সনিস্টের সাহায্য নিন

Haddii aad buuxinta foomkan doonay so in lagaa caawiyo,
fadlan la hadal soo dhaweynia barta takhartarkaaga.

假如閣下需要協助填寫這份表格，請與診所內的款接員聯絡。

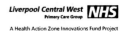

Liverpool Central West **NHS**
Primary Care Group

A Health Action Zone Innovations Fund Project

Help us to help you...

Important information required by your Doctor

Dear

Your Doctor's Surgery is working to make services better for all.

By answering the questions in this form you will be helping us to deliver better services to you as an individual. Your Doctor's Surgery will also get a better picture of the local population. This will help in planning new services and changing existing ones. You do not have to fill in this form but if you do, you will be helping us to help you.

The information you provide will be treated in the strictest confidence. Only staff here at your Surgery will use individual information. Information you give will be treated in the same way as other information we hold. When used in the planning of services all names and other identifying details will be removed.

Just post the form back to us in the freepost envelope or drop it into the Surgery. If you have any queries please contact the Surgery and we will answer your questions.

Thank you for your help -

❑ Please tick this box if you would like an opportunity to receive feedback on this work and/or become part of a patient participation group.

❑ I do not wish to fill this form in.

If your name, address or telephone number have changed from those printed on the front, please write in the correct details in the space provided below. **IMPORTANT - only do this if the details have changed.**
Remember, if you need any help to fill this in just ask the receptionist or the linkworker at your doctor's.

First Name: .... Surname: ....

House Number: .... Street: .... Postcode: .... Telephone: ....

Please think back over the last 12 months about how your health has been *compared to people of your own age*. How would you describe your health over the last 12 months?

😊 ❑ Excellent   🙂 ❑ Good   😐 ❑ Fair   🙁 ❑ Poor   ☹ ❑ Very Poor   😕 ❑ Not Sure

Figure 4.1   An example of a data collection form

How would you describe your religion?

☐ None   ☐ Christianity   ☐ Church of England   ☐ Roman Catholic   ☐ Buddhism   ☐ Hinduism
☐ Jehovah's Witness   ☐ Islam   ☐ Judaism   ☐ Sikhism
☐ Other Christian - write in: .... ☐ Other Religion - write in: ....

Are you a carer i.e. do you look after a friend or relative who is sick, disabled, elderly, has mental health problems or for any other reason?   ☐ Yes   ☐ No

Are you cared for i.e. do you have a friend or relative who helps you live your day to day life?
☐ Yes   ☐ No

If you have answered yes to either of these questions the surgery will contact you for more information

In which Country were you born?

☐ Bangladesh   ☐ China   ☐ Czech Republic   ☐ Egypt   ☐ England   ☐ Ghana
☐ Hong Kong   ☐ India   ☐ Iran   ☐ Iraq   ☐ Ireland   ☐ Libya
☐ Malaysia   ☐ Nigeria   ☐ Northern Ireland   ☐ Pakistan   ☐ Scotland   ☐ Somalia
☐ Wales   ☐ Yemen   ☐ Other, please write in: ....

How would you describe your Ethnic Group?

☐ Asian Bangladeshi   ☐ Asian Indian   ☐ Asian Other   ☐ Asian Pakistani   ☐ Black African
☐ Black Caribbean   ☐ Black Other   ☐ Chinese   ☐ Mixed Other   ☐ Mixed White & Asian
☐ Mixed White & Black African   ☐ Mixed White & Black Caribbean   ☐ Somali
☐ White British   ☐ White Irish   ☐ White Other   ☐ Yemeni
☐ Other, please write in: ....

What is your Main Spoken Language?

☐ Arabic   ☐ Bengali   ☐ Cantonese   ☐ Czech   ☐ English   ☐ French   ☐ Hakka
☐ Hindi   ☐ Mandarin   ☐ Polish   ☐ Portuguese   ☐ Punjabi   ☐ Russian   ☐ See-yip
☐ Somali   ☐ Spanish   ☐ Tamil   ☐ Urdu   ☐ Other, please write in: ....

Do you need an Interpreter/Translator   ☐ Yes   ☐ No

Do you use   ☐ British Sign Language   ☐ Lip Reading   ☐ A Loop System   ☐ Textphone/Minicom

What language do you prefer to read?

☐ Arabic   ☐ Bengali   ☐ Braille   ☐ Chinese   ☐ Czech   ☐ English   ☐ French
☐ Hindi   ☐ Polish   ☐ Portuguese   ☐ Punjabi   ☐ Russian   ☐ Somali   ☐ Spanish
☐ Tamil   ☐ Urdu   ☐ I do not read any languages

☐ Other, please write in: ....

Figure 4.1   Continued

In Liverpool training is supported by a direct line to a 'patient profiling officer' who can answer patients' questions in more detail, in addition to reference information that is left in practices. In general primary care practices that have developed patient profiling in different parts of the country have found that the collection of ethnicity data has not been as problematic as they had anticipated and patients have been willing to respond.

How should data be collected?

A method of data collection must be decided. Some have used opportunistic collection—for example, patients are handed a form to complete in reception as they attend the surgery. This has the advantage of being cheaper in the short term, but becomes less effective in the long term. Data accrues too slowly to be immediately useful. The impetus generated by staff training rapidly fades when they see diminishing return for their time investment. This sort of opportunistic approach is probably best used in addition to more proactive data collection (see below) and to sustain collection in the long term.

Our recommended alternative is to mail forms to patients. This is more expensive but provides more information more quickly. There are many ways of approaching a mailshot. Seek advice from the mail service. Schemes such as 'Mailsort' and 'Tailor Made Incentives' can significantly reduce mailing costs. Local departments that administer cervical cytology or child immunization letters can also advise, and possibly contract for the work. There are data protection issues in using an external agency to mail out a form to patients, but these may be overcome if the local PCT Caldicott committee approval is sought. The alternative is a manual mailshot using addresses obtained from practices clinical systems or PCT registers (Exeter systems).

There are several ways to maximize response rate:

♦ Forms can be labelled with each patient's name and address, addressed from individual GPs and printed with the NHS logo.

♦ If data is available on the languages spoken by the population, information about how to fill in the forms can be included in other languages. This information may be extrapolated from Exeter system data on country of birth, local knowledge of practice staff or interpreting services.

Experience around the country indicates most practices can expect around a third of their patients to respond to a first mailing.

Translation of the entire patient profiling form into another language is problematic. Cost, the inability to target forms without existing information on language requirements (chicken and egg situation) and the problems of translation of patients' answers when data is collated make this unfeasible.

Database templates

It is necessary to create a template for easy data entry and subsequent use of data. However, data storage on different primary care clinical systems can be a problem. Creating READ codes can be time consuming. The process for submitting new codes to the NHS Coding and Classification Centre (NHSCCC) – the guardians of the READ codes – can be unwieldy. When the NHSCCC will not create a code (e.g. for a non-standard ethnic group) only certain primary care system suppliers (e.g. EMIS and Meditel, but not IPS VAMP) will allow you to create a local code. Primary Care Trust IT departments should be able to create a template, as can various private companies or system suppliers if necessary. However, the 2001 Census ethnic categories and their READ codes will often be the best starting point. Initiatives around the country have already developed their own templates, which can be transferred from one site to another (see 'Further information'). It is likely that other sites may already have the basis for a template that can be adapted.

Benefits of patient profiling

Our experience is that preparation for patient profiling has provided those working in primary care with welcome and timely opportunities to discuss issues related to the health of BME and other communities. This, on its own, has initiated action to improve services in one practice which decided to employ a bilingual receptionist as a result.

Discussion with local community groups and voluntary organizations about the purpose of patient profiling has led to useful joint working on issues raised, for example identifying and tackling the high smoking prevalence in the Yemeni community in Liverpool. Local academic institutions may also be keen to work on issues arising from the information obtained. In Liverpool a closer relationship has formed between public health professionals and primary care teams and is developing further in new PCTs. Some specific examples of how the information collected in Liverpool has been used are outlined in Box 4.1.

Barriers to be overcome

Some funding is required, but need not be extensive. Harnessing community pressure and focusing on the equality agenda in current policy imperatives may help to facilitate the necessary resources. This currently non-statutory and innovative work may easily slip down the priority list for busy practices. By ensuring that a PCT or a dedicated 'patient profiler' is able to initiate the bulk of the early work (e.g. mailing forms, data entry and analysis), this can be avoided.

A lack of capacity in primary care to effectively use profiling data can be a problem. However, it can also be an opportunity to make better use of IT

Box 4.1 **Actions and service development following patient profiling in Liverpool**

- Identifying a high prevalence of smoking among a Yemeni practice population, who were also shown to be at high risk of heart disease and diabetes. This was borne out by discussions with members of the Yemeni community. This has led to an action research initiative in response.
- Identifying a need to fund a Yemeni community development worker.
- Information in appropriate languages has been sent to patients with history of stroke or epilepsy about services offered by the local neurological centre as part of its outreach work into the community.
- Practices have organized Somali and Yemeni and Bengali Health Days, which were well attended and popular with local communities. Practices invited all patients in appropriate languages, advertised within the local communities.
- One male single-handed practice with over 50% of its patients found to be from BME communities enlisted the support of the local PCT to recruit two bilingual receptionists and a female GP.
- A practice where 40% of patients were from BME groups was able to alter its appointment system to cater more effectively for patients whose first language was not English by initiating a same day appointment service with special arrangements, including 15-minute appointment slots, for patients needing interpreters.
- Practices are informing patients of the diabetes outreach in the community service, about the local multicultural diabetes project and health link workers.
- A PCT has produced leaflets in various languages about cervical smears and is targeting cervical smear defaulters from BME groups with information in appropriate languages.
- A PCT is conducting an 'equity of care audit', tracking patients with angina through the system from presentation in primary care through to specialist tertiary care.
- In some practices information is now recorded for individual patients on template referral letters about religion, language spoken and need for interpreter.

systems in primary care. Moreover, this can be a way of involving practices in the more population-based approach asked of PCTs and enable them to realize the benefits of accurate and systematic data recording.

The major barrier to patient profiling is a view that it is a special initiative for specific groups. The idea that this work is only relevant for practices with large BME communities is wrong. It is arguably even more relevant in practices with small BME populations, as staff have less experience dealing with non-English speakers and non-standard health needs. The new Race Relations Amendment Act (2000) placing a statutory duty on services to promote equality and patient profiling has been endorsed by the Commission for Racial Equality. This should help this crucial work to be mainstreamed and its benefits to spread throughout the health service.

Key points

- Patient profiling is essential for the development of services that respond effectively to ethnic and other diversity
- Patient profiling is not a special initiative for specific groups
- A solely opportunistic approach to data collection is not recommended
- Staff and community involvement is essential
- Liaison with other initiatives will reduce costs and make the process easier
- Creating a culture of using the data from the outset is vital
- Early demonstration of benefit to practices and patients is recommended

Acknowledgments

We would like to thank the Department of Health for initial funding, Liverpool Central Primary Care Trust for its continuing support, and Bennett Lee and Taher Qassim for being themselves.

Further information

Race Relations (amendment) Act 2000.
Disability Discrimination Act 1995.
Statutory Code of Practice on the duty to promote race equality (consultation draft). Commission for Racial Equality, 2001.
Smaje C, Le Grand J. Ethnicity, equity and the use of health services in the British NHS. *Social Science and Medicine* 1997; 45: 3485–3496.
Heath I. The role of ethnic monitoring in general practice. *British Journal of General Practice* 1991; 41: 310–311.
Delivering the NHS plan to diverse communities. London: NHS Executive, 2001.
Lee B, Gardner K, Jones B, Qassim T. *Ethnicity profiling in primary care, a Princes Park Model.* Liverpool: Public Health Sector, John Moores University, 2000. A report of ethnicity profiling at Princes Park Health Centre, Liverpool is available online at *http://www.nwpho.org.uk* or *http://www.ethnichealth-northwest.net*
http://www.doh.gov.uk/ethnicity2001guidance/index.htm provides guidance in collecting ethnic group data.
Ethnic monitoring. A guide for public authorities. London: Commission for Racial Equality, 2002. Available online at *http://www.cre.gov.uk*
Minority Ethnic Health mailing list: *http:/www.jiscmail.ac.uk/lists/minority-ethnic-health.html*

5 Improving access to health care

Rhian Loudon

Improving access to health care must mean improving access to services of quality that have a positive effect on health. As Chapter 3 has highlighted, access to care for people from black and minority ethnic groups (BMEGs) can be reduced, perpetuating inequity and disadvantage.[1] This can result from obvious deficiencies such as lack of bilingual support for effective communication. However, more subtle exclusion mechanisms can operate which may be more difficult to address (see Box 5.1).

In this chapter I discuss factors that may influence access to services and then provide some practical suggestions that readers may wish to consider. Many of the points raised here will underscore those from other chapters in this

---

Box 5.1   **Examples of subtle exclusion from effective care**

- *Equating 'use' with 'effective use' of a service.* For example, an elderly Gujarati-speaking Kenyan may seek the help of a GP for memory problems. The patient has ready access to his GP. Yet culturally appropriate tests of cognitive impairment may not be available, so the effectiveness of care may be less for the Kenyan patient than for others.
- *The absence of economic evaluations of interventions to improve access for people from BMEGs.*[2] This may mean that where economic efficiency is the most valued outcome measure, any arguments for initiatives to improve access for people from BMEGs lack force.
- *Gaps in research may not be filled because of uncritical acceptance of existing practice and value judgements.* For example people who do not speak English are routinely excluded from clinical research trials because they may be seen as too difficult to include (e.g. they require translated information). In contrast, huge effort may be made to meet the challenges of participants receiving different types of intervention or treatment in a trial.
- *Institutional racism.* For example, resources for services may be allocated in 'the way they always have' rather than based on an assessment of need. A study of community nursing found nurses working in inner city areas had larger patient populations (with people from BMEGs) than those working in more affluent areas. The *status quo* persisted because it was easier for the service not to change and there was no 'evidence' about how to allocate resources other than historically.[3]

book especially those relating to quality of care, patient profiling, effective communication, interpreting and advocacy, and learning to respond to diversity (Chapters 3, 4, 6, 7, 8 and 10).

Access and identity

Ethnicity is just one way of categorizing people. It is important to recognize that many of the issues for improving access to care are common to everyone. It is contentious just how dominant the 'ethnic' aspect of an individual's identity may be in shaping access to the health care system compared to other aspects of one's identity (such as socio-economic background) and indeed the identity of service providers (such as health professional status).

For example, which individual factor predominates in determining ability to access services when a person's ethnicity is combined with possession of private health insurance or educational level, or indeed the nature of the illness for which one is seeking treatment? Moreover, how might the characteristics, ethnic or otherwise, of the person from whom one has sought help influence access to care?

If people are divided up in ways other than ethnicity, for example able bodied and disabled, rich and poor, sighted and visually impaired then it can be seen that factors other than ethnicity may become more pertinent for an individual in a particular setting in determining his or her appropriate access to services.

Some of these issues are discussed elsewhere in this volume, for example in Chapters 15, 18 and 20 which deal with how age or refugee status or having cancer may combine with ethnicity and influence health and access to health care. However, despite this inevitable variation for each individual, there are also important aspects of services for populations and communities that are likely to disadvantage people from BMEGs and these are now considered.

The interaction of user and provider

The varying characteristics of health professionals, services and individual patients will all interact to influence the success of a service in improving health outcomes. Thus focusing solely on improving service structure will not ameliorate all problems.

Considerations for improving access will differ according to the context for care. A focus on widening access to the 7-minute 'routine' GP-patient consultation held in surgery hours will ignore the variety of interactions that a patient may have in a primary care setting. For example, different professional perspectives will be brought to bear in interactions between patients and, say, GPs, health visitors or pharmacists. The setting for the interaction may be an out-of-hours service, a screening service or chronic illness clinic. Patients may perceive their problem as urgent or routine.

All these factors will present specific challenges for patient access. In what follows I have chosen a selection of roles and responsibilities that those working in primary care may adopt that might illustrate some general points to improve access in practice.

Equal opportunities and employment practice

Rewarding bilingual workers appropriately

People who speak both a community language and English can be a great asset to, say, a general practice. If such skills are to be sought with qualifications or tests of ability then they should be valued appropriately and in salary. For example, not only will access to services be improved by employing a bilingual receptionist, but the importance attached to communication between staff and patients will be underlined.

Recruiting staff

If a practice wishes to recruit staff who reflect the characteristics of the local population then it should advertise appropriately. In addition to placing adverts in local English language newspapers, putting adverts in local black and minority ethnic group (BMEG) language publications or using different informal networks such as local community workers or advocates will help. The Commission for Racial Equality highlights the importance of notifying vacancies to job centres, careers offices, schools and colleges attended by people from BME groups.

Tackling racial harassment

The 2000 Amendment to the 1976 Race Relations Act means for the first time that public services, including primary care practices, will have to demonstrate that they are working for equality rather than merely avoiding discrimination. Formulating an effective equal opportunities policy may help practices consider their response to racial discrimination perceived either on the part of patients by staff, or of staff to each other, or of patients towards staff.

Difficulty in providing an equitable service available to all may arise when responding to racist abuse of staff by patients. For example if a practice is actively considering removing a patient from a practice list, perhaps for a limited period, because they have shouted racial abuse at a member of staff, then clearly this patient is being judged to have forfeited the right to care from this practice. If staff from BMEGs are to feel valued then they must feel that an appropriate response is made when they are abused by others. Clearly these are sensitive judgements to make. The implications of such a decision may be very different in an urban area with alternative options for GP registration and a rural setting with only one practice for the locality.

Staff training

Professional education and training that includes all those working in primary care is vital in developing an accessible and effective service (see Chapter 10). Beyond the importance of responding to individuals with 'cultural sensitivity', the wider roles of primary care workers in ameliorating disadvantage and widening access merit debate (see Box 5.2).

Box 5.2   A dilemma for a GP

You think your practice doesn't receive a fair enough share of district nursing services in your Primary Care Trust (PCT) area to offer effective care for your patients who include people from BMEGs. What should you do?

Possible actions and their possible consequences

A   Take some research evidence such as that referred to above in Box 5.1[3] to the next public meeting of your PCT. Inform the local press and any local BME community groups of your intentions, and get them to come along. Challenge the PCT board to develop an action plan to correct years of inequity.

- *Pros:* PCT board need to appear willing to listen and seen to be working for equal opportunities. Cause will be publicized and may attract supporters.
- *Cons:* Absence of local data to your support argument. PCT board may feel threatened and unprepared. The need for action over this issue may be downgraded by arguments over other perceived injustices. Potential supporters may be alienated by a public and potentially acrimonious debate.

B   Write to the PCT board quoting the research paper and its findings, draw appropriate local parallels and ask for their response.

- *Pros:* Gives time for considered response. Board can develop an action plan that uses local circumstances to effect change.
- *Cons:* Board may feel no external pressure to alter the status quo given the priorities competing for their attention.

C   Disseminate findings to local district nurses, GPs and patients and arrange a meeting to decide on a collective plan of action. Present this to PCT board.

- *Pros:* Potentially establish a commitment to change from all parties ('stakeholders'). Could lead to collection of local data to support arguments. Develop a workable plan of action that is owned by those who will put it into practice.
- *Cons:* Potential for variation among participants in familiarity with research methods and skills at interpreting evidence. Potential for disagreement about whether inequities are due to resource allocation or poor individual professional practice. Individual behaviour change or educational strategies may be suggested as an alternative to tackling funding issues. Fortuitously the suggested strategies do not affect those present at the meeting.

D   Make a conscious effort to think whether a patient would benefit from district nurse input during each consultation and if appropriate make a referral in line with patient preference.

- Pros: This is 'patient centred care.' Avoids time-consuming negotiation with PCT. Takes responsibility for one's own practice and leaves decisions about the parameters within which one operates to someone else.
- Cons: Ignores a public health function and advocacy role of you as a GP. Your district nurse colleagues may be unable to cope with a potential increase in referrals with no matching increase in resources, so standards fall. This increases staff sickness rates or turnover.

As the potential disadvantages arising from action D in Box 5.2 may show, many health professionals are very familiar with the experience of what happens when high expectation meets inadequate resource. Often the first thing that happens is that a bad situation gets worse and existing staff become demoralized. However, these issues should be considered in staff training. Consider what strategies for change are possible? What are the advantages and disadvantages for different patient groups of such strategies?

Reviewing practice systems

Privacy and confidentiality

As discussed in Chapter 7, the routine acceptance by staff and patients of bringing a relative or friend to act as an interpreter may need to be challenged. If a practice is committed to providing a confidential and private service, then the onus is on practice staff to ask individual patients if they require an interpreter when making an appointment rather than waiting until the time of the consultation itself. Similarly, practices can proactively publicize the availability of local interpreting and advocacy services, and indeed any language skills of its staff in practice leaflets, notices and tapes that describe the services provided by the practice.

New patient registration

The process of registering new patients in general practice can be used as an opportunity for patients to ask about the structure and role of local services as well as services provided by an individual practice. This may also be a good opportunity to conduct patient profiling (see Chapter 4).

Prolonged absence overseas

Practices might consider the provision they make for people embarking on a prolonged absence overseas. This might typically be a visit of 2–3 months to relatives, which is common for example among some South Asian families. Conventionally NHS prescriptions for repeat medications are provided for only 1 month when patients are out of the UK. However, depending on the nature of their terms of service, GPs might prescribe additional quantities of medication on private prescriptions for those patients who are uncertain if they will be able to obtain their normal medication at their destination. This possibility might be raised when people attend for travel vaccinations. Similarly, any effect on childhood immunization schedules can be anticipated and alternative arrangements made.

Gender

Gender may or may not be important for an individual (of any ethnicity) in determining whether they seek help for a particular problem or attend, for example, for a screening procedure. However, practices need to consider how much choice patients are offered in terms of the gender of staff who provide services, how that gender mix is reflected in day-to-day appointments and how that information is publicized. A practice policy for chaperones during patient examination is helpful. Some practices offer a waiting area that allows for self-segregation by gender for those who wish it. Staff should also be encouraged to reflect on how their gender, age, ethnicity and so on may influence their interactions and examinations with patients (see Chapter 10).

Working across health services

Much research has explored inequities in the use of health care services by people from different groups in Britain.[2,4] Ethnicity-related research has been compromised by not adequately considering socio-economic status, differing levels of morbidity, and health 'needs'. In general, BME populations are likely to consult GPs more than majority groups. Use of hospital out-patient services tends to be less for BMEGs in lower age groups but equivalent or greater in older age groups. As noted in Box 5.1, counts of service use cannot be used as evidence that people's needs are being met.

It remains to be seen if opportunities arising from the reorganization of primary care services may address issues such as resource allocation to areas of disadvantage and more appropriate and creative integration of services. However, thinking about the point of referral to hospital services, as a minimum GPs can usefully identify and highlight in referral letters any need for interpreting services to be provided, or whether a patient has a gender preference. Standard advice about what to do if an appointment fails to materialize could also be reiterated to patients. Accordingly, PCTs might wish to write into their service level agreements with other NHS Trusts that a service will be provided in a language of the patient's choosing using an interpreter as appropriate.

Similarly, primary care workers may wish to review their own practice and consider whether they are offering the full range of services for all their patients. For example, is cognitive behavioural therapy considered for all? Lessons might also be gained from others, for example speech and language therapists or physiotherapists, about how they have dealt with particular issues, such as lack of shared spoken language in their clinical practice

Some lessons from real life

Establishing interpreting services

The advent of PCTs can make a big difference to the availability of interpreting services. In one large city, for example, an overstretched interpreting service for all localities collapsed as its budget was overspent. However, as practitioners within a PCT recognized the importance of interpreting services in sustaining a meaningful and equitable service and meeting local priorities, additional financial provision was made available to allow the service to continue.

Conflicting priorities

Patient priorities may be different to those of health professionals. For example, a woman attended a GP surgery having made a routine appointment with the one female doctor in a practice, with whom she did not share a common language. In the limited language that was shared the doctor offered to arrange for a free, professional interpreter to be present at a follow-up appointment. The patient declined and went back to the waiting room and asked if any of the waiting patients would act as interpreter for her. One woman came forward to do so and the consultation proceeded and appeared to conclude in a satisfactory way for the patient, for a problem that in the doctor's view was relatively minor.

Helpful resources

The Commission for Racial Equality (see 'Further information') has developed useful materials for primary care practices that they might find useful when formulating equal opportunities policies, thinking about employment practices and considering principles of fairness in the way they offer services and work with patients. These materials include examples of the basic components of a race equality policy; educational strategies for practice staff and the legal framework for positive action.

Conclusion

Thinking about improving access to services for people from BMEGs and the specific yet subtle ways in which disadvantage may be perpetuated generates general principles for health care. These can be applied for everyone, in particular to improve access for other disadvantaged groups.

Key points

- Ethnicity is just one aspect of an individual's identity that may influence access to health care
- Patient identity, service and health professional characteristics interact to determine ease of access
- Mechanisms that perpetuate disadvantage may be subtle
- Rates of service use are not equivalent to rates of access to treatment or positive health outcomes

♦ Over or under use of services by groups with equal need may reflect a poor quality service: identification can be a stimulus to further study and change

References

1. Smaje C. Explaining patterns of utilisation. In: *Health, 'Race' and Ethnicity*. London: King's Fund, 1995, pp. 100–113 (a useful summary of research to 1995 and a thoughtful discussion of the issues).
2. Atkinson M, Clark M, Clay D, Johnson M, Owen D, Szczepura A. *Systematic review of ethnicity and health service access for London*. Coventry: Centre for Health Service Studies, Warwick Business School, University of Warwick, 2001 (a recent literature review that makes recommendations on the evidence needed from future research).
3. Gerrish K. Inequalities in service provision: an examination of institutional influences on the provision of district nursing care to minority ethnic communities. *Journal of Advanced Nursing* 1999; 30: 1263–1271 (an ethnographic study that discusses the subtle ways in which unequal provision may be sustained and the difficulties faced when trying to change the status quo).
4. Goddard M, Smith P. *Equity of access to health care*. University of York: Centre for Health Economics, 1998 (a useful summary and commentary).

Further information

Griffiths C, Kaur G, Gantley M, Feder G, Hillier S, Goddard J. Influences on hospital admission for asthma in south Asian and white adults: qualitative interview study. *BMJ* 2001; 323: 1–8 (this study highlights the complex mix of factors that affect access to good quality health care such as organisation, attitudes of staff and patients, power relationships and partnership models of care).
Commission for Racial Equality website: *http://www.cre.gov.uk*

6 Effective cross-cultural communication

Jon Fuller

This chapter deals with communication between people from diverse ethnic groups and health professionals. Of course, we all have our own ethnicities and cultural influences (see Chapter 10). Thus all health encounters are 'cross-cultural'. Although there are some challenges posed by particular differences between people, the principles of effective communication discussed here are applicable to all patient–professional consultations.

By becoming a 'professional', the doctor, nurse or other health professional puts a barrier between themselves and the patient. The greater the difference, the more difficult it is for the professional to put themselves in the patient's position, to empathize fully, to see them as human beings in their cultural context, or to see a situation from their patient's point of view.

Developing the right approach

Attaining effective communication is a skill, which can be learned and improved by training. Nevertheless, training alone is not sufficient. For tennis players to reach the top, they work on their technique, but they know that they will not achieve great heights unless they also have the right attitudes to complement these skills. The same is true of consulting in health care settings where there are differences of any kind. The right attitudes include acceptance of the relevance of others' beliefs, cultural sensitivity, and an awareness of your own prejudices (see Chapter 10).

There are numerous examples where challenges can arise: for example people with alcohol problems, teenagers with second unwanted pregnancies, or 'heartsink' patients. To consult to the greatest benefit, the health professional must develop some degree of understanding of the patient's perspective.

> Sometimes when I am faced with a new patient, I want them to get on with it, and let me get on and see the next patient. But as their story unfolds, my attitude to them changes, I start to see them in a more humane way, somehow more human, and therefore more deserving of my attention.
> [inner-city GP]

Sometimes it is clear there are difficulties in the consultation. This can be for very practical reasons, such as language differences, or it becomes obvious that health professional and patient are just not on the same wavelength. Sometimes the health professional will not be aware of the degree of their own ignorance, and that their assumptions are wrong. It is important to:

◆ attempt to understand the patient's point of view, their background and their understanding of the problem

◆ remember that you will often make assumptions about patient's beliefs, understanding, previous experience and perceived needs that may be completely erroneous.

These might seem mundane points. However, in the hurly-burly of appointments systems, over-running consultations, difficult decisions and language differences, they are often forgotten. Time in health care systems is a rare commodity. But the greater the cultural difference between health professional and patient, the more time for reflection is needed.

Expectations of patient and professional

Everyone has a history. The problem is that in communicating we are often unaware of the effect of our own history and forget that the other person has one too. This is equally true of health professionals and patients. The effect of this history is expressed in our stereotypes, prejudices, and most importantly in our expectations of the consultation. Very often the expectations of the health professional and the patient of the consultation are at odds, creating problems. It is worth examining the many influences on the expectations of both health professional and patient. These include personal experience, previous experience of health care, explanations for illness and pre-existing stereotypes.

Previous personal experience

Of course, previous experiences of health care and illness have a very powerful influence on expectations. It might be said that much of a professional's education is based on their experience and their learning from that experience. Similarly, patients will have a background of their own experiences or those of family and friends who have been in similar situations. Where patients (or the influential adults in their family or cultural group) have been brought up in a different culture, it is inevitable that their personal experiences will differ from that of the health professional.

Previous experiences of the health care system

Patients who have experienced a different health care system often have different expectations from the health professional. For example, in contrast to the

UK, in other countries it might be considered the norm for a patient to see a number of physicians or specialists for opinions about one condition rather than a single GP, or to attend a consultation with several family members.

> You must remember that where I come from in Turkey, it is normal to see more than one doctor about an illness, if you can afford it.
> [Turkish bilingual health advocate]

Patients and professionals have their own experience of how health care systems work, which is often coloured by their knowledge about how it should work. How much their view of the system fits with reality may vary.

Explanations for illness

The term 'health beliefs' is often used to describe an individual's (or cultural group's) understanding of the process of maintaining health or becoming ill. This assumes that each individual has a coherent, complete and stable model for their health. The reality is that an individual's understanding of health is usually incomplete, sometimes contradictory, and alters to fit each situation they find themselves in.

It is preferable to think in terms of an individual's explanations for illness. Health professionals have their own explanatory system readily to hand, although their explanations may not be as evidence-based as first appears. The explanations that patients bring may be relatively inaccessible to the health professional.

Patients may be reluctant to expose their beliefs to the scrutiny of the health professional. They may believe that it is not their role to discuss their own views, and not the health professional's role to ask ('it is the doctor's job to find out what is wrong with me, that's what I came for'). They may not have had the experience of presenting their thoughts about their health to a health professional before.

Stereotypes

Stereotyping and prejudice, defined in Chapter 10, are important influences on communication. Everyone stereotypes others and may hold prejudices. It is important to be aware of their existence and what they are. In this way it is possible to take them into account, albeit imperfectly, in our communication with others.

> I consulted a number of times with a Turkish patient (with ischaemic heart disease). He was extremely obsequious, thanking me profusely for the slightest thing in a way that I found almost unpleasant, 'un English' I suppose. Talking to a Turkish advocate he told me that people from the patient's area do tend to be very polite. Somehow this helped me see the patient as behaving normally rather than unpleasantly grovelling.
> [GP]

People's accents are a powerful determinant of stereotyping. As well as a source of jokes, assumptions are made based on the degree the accent varies from that of 'educated and intelligent society'. In the USA, for example, people with accents from the southern states tend to be assumed to be less intelligent than those with an accent associated with northern states. Of course health professionals should remember that patients will also have their own set of stereotypes and prejudices about the professional and the health care system, especially if this is a first meeting.

Conflicting expectations

Bochner[1] has divided the potential sources of confusion within cross-cultural interactions into four types:

+ *Role confusion* occurs when either health professional or patient (or occasionally both) do not understand what is expected of them.

  A patient from West Africa came to see me after flying in from there. He said he felt unwell, probably because of being delayed in his travel. I agreed, unsure what he wanted from me. After some time he asked me for malaria tablets. After further history and examination he turned out to have malaria. Afterwards I asked him why he had not told me he thought he had malaria. He replied that he did not realize he could have done so.
  [GP]

+ *Role disparity* takes place when patient and professional disagree with each other about their roles.

  I become irritated by people who come to see me to ask for referral to a specialist for things I feel I can deal with myself. This often happens with patients who originate from countries where primary care is not as prominent as in the UK.
  [GP]

+ *Definition disparity* happens when people disagree about the definition of an event, the cause, the implications or the meaning.

  When I first started working in my practice we had a lot of patients from Nigeria. Sometimes fit looking young men would come in and complain that they had 'whole body weakness'. I used to find this very irritating and contrary to the evidence before me, and then I realized that this was just their way of saying 'I do not feel very well'.
  [East London GP]

+ *Goal disparity* is where health professional and patient have different aims for the consultation.

  I have one patient, an asylum seeker, with housing problems and difficulties in his relationship with his teenage children. He comes to me regularly complaining of headaches. He is insistent that he has a severe physical problem and demands increasingly strong medications, I am insistent that his headaches originate from his very difficult situation and am insistent on trying to deal with his problems.
  [GP]

These sources of confusion arise because of differing expectations and factors that shape them. They can be further influenced by other aspects of communication outlined below.

Non-verbal communication

It has been suggested that in a normal conversation the verbal component may carry less than a third of the social meaning of a situation, and more than two thirds is conveyed non-verbally. Health professionals and patients may misinterpret each other if the non-verbal communication they use, for example gestures, touch, proximity, head and body movements are based on different cultural conventions.

Use of some facial expressions seem to be common worldwide, for example a smile means happiness and a frown the opposite almost everywhere. Although the degree to which these expressions are employed may be culture specific, a welcoming smile seems rarely likely to hinder and often helps. Other forms of non-verbal communication can have different meanings. Perhaps the most important is degree of eye contact. In some cultural groups looking the other person in the eye is a sign of honesty; in others it can be a sign of disrespect, particularly between gender or age groups.

Para-verbal communication

Para-verbal communication includes politeness conventions, how information is delivered, including degrees of directness, tone of voice, stress on words and phrases, pace and use of silence.

Different language groups have different politeness conventions. A good example is the use of 'please' and 'thank you'. These words appear less commonly in some language groups, for example South Asian and Scandinavian languages. They therefore tend not to be used so much when those whose first language is one of the South Asian or Scandinavian languages speak in English, which can lead to perceptions of abruptness or rudeness when they talk to English speakers.

Similarly the degree of directness used by different language speakers can clash. English-English speakers tend to be relatively indirect, whereas African-Caribbean-, West African-English and South Asian-English speakers tend to be more direct. The effect may make the former appear deceitful to the latter (never saying what they mean), and the latter may be perceived as aggressive to the former.

These differences, and those in tone, stress, pace and use of silence, can lead to misinterpretation of motive. They can affect whether information is to be believed and what actions should be taken. Churchill reportedly said that the

Americans and the English are divided by the same language. They are not the only ones!

Where language is not shared

So far this chapter has assumed that the health professional and patient at least share a language, even if they do not share the way it is delivered. Clearly when language is not shared, or is only partially shared effective communication may be difficult and much can be lost. At best, practical and clinical issues might be dealt with, while psychosocial issues or information concerning health promotion and disease prevention remain unaddressed. At worst, this can lead to misdiagnosis, inappropriate treatment or worse.

The crucial importance of health professionals working with and valuing bilingual colleagues, such as interpreters, link workers and advocates is discussed in Chapters 7 and 8. However, communication in this context can still be improved, depending on the skill of the health professional.

Defer the consultation?

First, consider whether it is necessary to continue a consultation where language is not shared, or whether it should be postponed until language assistance can be obtained. There is often a tendency to continue the consultation regardless. This may be unavoidable in a critically urgent situation, but it is often better to wait until help with communication can be arranged.

Reduce anxiety and remember the basics

It is particularly important to keep the atmosphere relatively relaxed. This may be hard to do, with the prospect of a frustrating consultation ahead. However, many patients enter the consultation feeling nervous, particularly when they do not share the language of the health professional, or are not confident speaking in the health professional's language. Thus their level of anxiety can increase, which may compromise their ability to communicate further.

Many professionals, perhaps because they are concentrating on understanding and being understood, can lose their basic communication skills which would encourage the patient to relax and be able to communicate. These include showing courtesy, interest and concern, allowing time, showing patience and using non-verbal reassurance.

Every attempt should be made to get the patient's name correct. It often helps to ask for the patient's assistance with pronunciation, and then make a note on their notes of how it is done. Continuity and follow-up is particularly important, first because the patient has started to learn how to communicate with that person, and secondly because there is much less for the patient to explain.

Attend to para-verbal communication

It is helpful to keep an even tone, not to speed up delivery and not to shout. It does not help to switch to 'pidgin', speaking in abbreviated 'easy' phrases. This is not necessarily easier for the patient and can be patronizing. It is helpful to bear in mind the normal para-verbal structure of the patient's cultural group. Try discussing this with someone who is bilingual and from that cultural group, if they are available.

As the consultation proceeds it is important to signal any change of subject to the patient. If the subject is switched without warning and the patient is hanging on to the thread of the discussion, there is a likelihood that they will become completely lost (this of course is also important when communicating with someone with hearing impairment).

Confirmation that the patient has understood information or instructions should be carried out by asking a question that does not require the answer 'yes'. The response 'yes' can mean 'I have understood correctly', or 'I do not quite understand, but I will go away and think about it' or even 'I do wish you would stop talking to me, I do not understand'. Similarly, do not take nods and other expressions at face value. It can be preferable to ask the patient to explain back to you what they have understood or what they are going to do.

Use other aids to communication

Communication can be much enhanced by using pictures, diagrams and mime to convey meaning. For instance, there are a number of pictorial aids that some health professionals use to help identify parts of the body. There are also health-oriented lists of words and their translations in different languages. Different health professionals find these of variable use.

It is worth writing down important points or giving patients other written material to take away, even if this is in English. Most people will have access to someone in their community who can translate. There are a number of health promotion and information leaflets available in different languages, but it is worth remembering that some older people from migrant communities are not literate in the written form of their language, and younger members of the community may be bilingual verbally but not in the written text of their mother tongue. The importance of using translated audiovisual material is obvious. These issues are discussed further in Chapter 3.

Finally, of course, health professionals can learn to speak some of the languages of the patients they meet. Even where learning may be confined to a few words of greeting or simple enquiry, it can send a message to the patient that the health professional respects and is interested in them. Moreover, it may offer humble acknowledgement of the professional's own linguistic limitations.

Key points

◆ Cross-cultural communication can be challenging but is a skill that can be improved

◆ Be aware of your stereotypes and prejudices

◆ You and your patients have expectations of the consultation that may not agree

◆ Your patient will have their own understanding of their condition, but this may be difficult to access

◆ Be aware of the effect of non-verbal and para-verbal communication on both yourself and your patient

Reference

1. Bochner S. *Cultures in contact: studies in cross cultural interaction.* Oxford: Pergamon, 1982.

Further information

Bradby H. Communication, interpretation and translation. In: Culley L, Dyson S (eds). *Ethnicity and nursing practice.* Basingstoke: Palgrave, 2001.

Fuller J, Toon P. *Medical practice in a multicultural society.* London: Heinemann, 1988.

Kai J. Cross-cultural communication. *Medicine* 2000; 28(10): 36–38.

Skelton J, Kai J, Loudon R. Cross-cultural communication in medicine: questions for educators. *Medical Education* 2001; 35: 257–261.

7 Interpreting and translation

David Jones and Paramjit Gill

It is obvious that high-quality health care requires effective communication between patient and health professional.[1] Recent demographic changes accompanying globalization have created urban areas in the UK with highly linguistically diverse populations. For example, over 300 different language groups of significant size have been identified in London alone.[2] Other cities and towns can boast language speakers in a similar range of languages. The evidence suggests that the proportion of non-English speakers remains high even when individuals have been resident in the UK for some time.[3]

The NHS was established before the period of greatest immigration into the UK, at a time when doctors could once have expected to share the same culture and language as their patients. This expectation has changed: minority ethnic groups comprise over 7% of the UK population (see Chapter 1). However, it is far from clear that the NHS has changed rapidly enough, especially in the inner cities, to meet the challenge posed when patients and health professionals may not be able to communicate adequately in a shared language.

Spectrum of language service provision

The language barrier challenge to health professionals and health service providers is felt globally. The response in terms of appropriate language support has been categorized[4] as ranging across a spectrum, from no provision to *ad hoc* provision to comprehensive provision.

Language barriers in health care can only be equitably and effectively overcome by comprehensive language service provision. This is defined as delivery of needed languages via a service supported by training and accreditation with broad principles of access established and followed by public sector and relevant private sector agencies.[4] The UK offers *ad hoc* provision, but often the experience of individual health professionals and patients may be of no provision with huge frustration and anxiety from the attendant language barrier.

Challenges for service development

The majority of initial health care contacts take place in general practice. GPs in inner cities may increasingly be able to obtain a professional interpreter for 'important' consultations, but what of consultations that are not planned in advance? Only practices with a majority of patients from a single language community can expect to have an interpreter available throughout surgery hours. The much more typical inner city practice, with small numbers of non-English speaking patients from several language communities, is likely to have very limited access to professional interpreting.

In the absence of patient profiling (Chapter 4), Primary Care Trusts (PCTs) lack knowledge about the languages spoken in their districts and of the extent of the need for interpreter services, which are generally not available outside traditional working hours. Inadequate resources devoted to communication and information services create a much-impaired service for patients from minority ethnic groups.

Doctors and other health care workers may struggle to provide adequate care but are thwarted by an institutional orientation towards a standard of language service provision no longer appropriate for a heterogeneous population.

Current models of language provision

Health professionals must, then, choose between several imperfect alternatives. Phelan and Parkman[5] have drawn attention to the disadvantage of using friends and relatives for interpreting in consultations and, in particular, the importance of not using children.

Children lack the emotional and cognitive maturity to assume the responsibility of interpreting conversations between parents and professionals. In many families details of bodily function and dysfunction are private and an unsuitable subject for discussion with children. Despite official acceptance that children are not appropriate interpreters for their parents, young children are often used as interpreters.

The lack of interpreting services for non-English speaking patients presenting acutely is a source of real danger for the patient and adds significantly to the stress experienced by the clinician and the informal interpreter.

Types of interpreter

Although it seems self-evident that effective communication in health care in the presence of a language barrier requires an adult interpreter, who should act as an interpreter?

The interpreter may be informal – perhaps a family member or friend or a bilingual health worker – or a formal interpreter who may or may not be trained specifically for work in a health care setting.

Some informal interpreters may achieve effective communication between patient and health professional. They are widely used in general practice, and represent an obvious and pragmatic response to a language barrier. However, there are a number of concerns. There is evidence from textual analysis that informal interpreters make more frequent errors than professional interpreters and that these errors include deletions and insertions which distort the meaning of the interpreted communication. There is also the well-documented tendency for informal interpreters to pursue and impose their own agenda rather than that of the patient.

The professional interpreter will have received adequate training which is specific both for the health care context of the NHS and for the cultural context of the individuals concerned. Thus the effectiveness and accuracy of the subsequent communication is likely to be enhanced.

In order to maintain and improve standards, a continuous process of evaluation involving written evaluation, oral feedback and periodic external evaluation is essential. This type of quality assurance of interpreting services is extremely rare within the NHS.

Working with an interpreter

How can we work most effectively with professional interpreters? Most attempts to overcome the language barrier between health professional and patient involve consecutive interpretation, where there is a pause while speech content is delivered in the second language.

There have been attempts in the USA to explore the use of simultaneous interpreting, using headsets in a similar way to their use in multilingual international conference settings. Consecutive interpreting can be delivered by a physically present (proximate interpreter) or by a remote interpreter via a telephone line or by teleconferencing. It is also important for frontline staff, such as receptionists, to have access to interpreting services so that they can explain arrangements for arranging an interpreter.

Within the consulting room many factors influence the extent to which successful communication can be achieved via an interpreter (see Box 7.1). A triangular seating arrangement allows the health professional to see and clearly communicate with both the interpreter and the patient.

Box 7.1 **Key points working with an interpreter**

- Check seating arrangements
- Speak directly to the patient
- Be aware of non-verbal communication
- Avoid jargon and figures of speech
- Check the patient's understanding
- Use written materials

It is important to try to speak directly to the patient, but the interpreter should be free to decide whether they feel more comfortable speaking in the first or third person.[6] Sensitivity to body language and non-verbal communication is essential to achieve the patient's trust and confidence.

Health professionals should avoid jargon and figures of speech. They should speak for a sentence or two before pausing to allow the interpreter to interpret what has been said. Interpreting in health care is difficult work, and interpreters may need to interrupt to seek clarification of a word or a concept or to request the health professional to speak more slowly.

Extra care is required when explaining procedures or the details of medication and arrangements for follow-up and review. To feel confident that adequate communication has been achieved, it may be necessary to repeat what has been said and to ask the patient to give their understanding of what has been agreed. Written materials translated into the patient's language can be very helpful in supporting the consultation (see below).

Interpreted consultations are inevitably longer than consultations between speakers of the same language. Despite the great time pressure under which most NHS health professionals work, it is extremely important at end of the consultation to ask the patient if there is anything they feel they have not understood or wish to discuss.

Guidelines on best practice in the use of interpreters already exist, but there is considerable evidence that they are ignored by many health professionals.[7] The relationship between guidelines and actual practice needs to be strengthened by adherence to locally agreed guidelines. An opportunity exists with the development of clinical governance (see Chapter 3) within PCTs for a tighter adherence by clinicians to good practice in the use of interpreters in the consultation.

Medico-legal issues

The presence of a language barrier raises important medico-legal issues. Clinicians who make a diagnosis without an adequate history open themselves to accusations of malpractice. It is part of good medical practice to record and inform your local NHS or PCT if your ability to treat patients safely is compromised by lack of interpreting provision.

Where there is no interpreter, or only extremely inadequate provision, health professionals acting without informed consent may find that they are vulnerable to legal action on the grounds of battery or assault. Treating patients without adequate language provision should be regarded as unethical except in an emergency.

Access and geography

The need to access health care may be urgent. There are rising pressures in primary care to ensure that patients are able to obtain even routine appointments within 48 hours. Professional interpreters will need to be available at short notice if the large UK population of non-English speakers is to have a service similar to that of the English-speaking majority population. The geographical distribution of non-English speakers means that access and geography are interlinked.

For example, it may be cost-effective to provide Bengali-speaking interpreters in every clinic and health centre and hospital outpatient department in East London (where a large Bengali-speaking population is concentrated). However, this is not an option when many more diverse language groups are present in a locality. For example, this is not a realistically affordable option for the speakers of extreme minority languages such as Yoruba or Serbo-Croat.

The 'sessional' solution, where a practice or other health service offers certain language services at specific times, say on designated afternoons each week can be superficially attractive. However, this effectively institutionalizes a second-rate and restricted service for a specific linguistic minority.

Remote access interpreting

Telephone interpreting (a 'language line') is more widely used in the USA and Australia where there is greater recognition that the need for rapid access and presence of linguistic diversity create a problem that can only be addressed by telephone interpreting services.

In the UK provision of telephone interpreting mirrors that of language service generally, in being patchy and *ad hoc*. It involves both patient and professional using a hands-free phone with an interpreter on the telephone line. Specific considerations are required (see Box 7.2).

A remote service may result in loss of potentially supportive face-to-face contact which may compromise communication of complex or sensitive information. However, it may sometimes help address embarrassment, or concerns about confidentiality, because the interpreters are unlikely to come from the same locality as the patient. Language line services in the UK cover over 100 different languages (www.languageline.co.uk).

Box 7.2 **Essentials of effective telephone interpreting**

- Call handling to ensure rapid contact
- Dedicated medical telephone interpreter
- Good-quality hands-free conference phone
- Appropriate desk positioning of conference phone
- Agreed protocols (e.g. use of patient's first name only – ensures that concerns about confidentiality (who is listening) are reduced
- Interpreting service and telephone charges free to health professionals

Towards a comprehensive interpreting service

This requires knowledge of the number and distribution of non-English speakers and of the languages spoken (Box 7.3). Although this information can be extrapolated from modified Census data this method is unsatisfactory. There remains an urgent requirement for data collection at local PCT and national level (see Chapter 4).

Any truly comprehensive service is likely to include the provision of a mix of physically present and remote interpreters.

Translation

The need to provide translated materials has the same context as the need to provide interpreting in health care. Literacy levels in different language communities may differ from national literacy levels in English. The finding of significant levels of illiteracy in any particular language should not be used to justify the failure to provide written material for those wishing and able to obtain more information about aspects of illness, health promotion or the availability of services.

As with interpreting, the provision of translated materials can range from nil to patchy provision of some literature in appropriate languages. As with interpreting, the aim of service providers should be comprehensive provision. Aspects of comprehensive provision of translated materials include:

♦ appropriate languages for local context
♦ broad range of materials, for example public notices/posters/letters to patients/ advice leaflets/prescriptions
♦ efficient system of access to materials and their re-supply.

Method of translation

There is no 'gold standard' describing the most appropriate method of translating materials for use in health care, and further research is needed. It remains

---

Box 7.3 **Key indicators of a successful delivery model**

♦ Matching of language resources to language need
♦ Ensuring rapid access and 24-hour availability
♦ Effective evaluation of quality and satisfaction with service delivery
♦ Ensuring affordability
♦ Appropriate training accreditation and equipment support
♦ Ensuring health workers and health providers follow established principles of access

important to remember that what is most required in adapting an information leaflet or poster by translation into another language is as accurate a restatement of meaning as possible, rather than linguistic precision.

This does not mean that a rigorous approach should not be adopted. Guidelines suggest undertaking several independent translations that are compared and back translated, followed by the testing of the acceptability of translations to the relevant patient group.

Improving provision

The provision of a comprehensive range of translated materials requires a strategic approach at regional and national level that has yet to be achieved. Despite this, much can be done locally at PCT level. Making translated material available at the point of delivery of health care requires organization and the use of appropriate technology. For example, the NHS net allows the potential to access a vast range of documents, including health information translated into several different languages. Desktop laser printers in the consulting room can be use to produce translated leaflets without the need to keep leaflet racks re-supplied.

Conclusion

The linguistic diversity of the UK population presents a huge challenge to a largely monolingual health service and to those who work in it. There is an understanding of what constitutes good practice and the technology now exists to deliver high-quality language services to every health care setting.

The political will to allocate greater resources to language services has yet to emerge. Health care practice without adequate communication due to language barriers is unsafe, unethical and discriminatory. The current unsatisfactory state of interpreting and translation provision needs to be challenged by health professionals and managers.

Key points

- The UK is linguistically diverse
- There is mismatch between need for and provision of effective interpreting
- Use of children as interpreters remains widespread and is not acceptable
- Formally trained interpreters offer advantages over family and friends
- The potential of 'remote' interpreting remains under-developed but expansion seems likely in the future
- Provision of translated material needs to be more readily accessible

References

1. Stewart MA. Effective physician-patient communication and health outcomes: a review. *Canadian Medical Association Journal* 1995; 152(9): 1423–1433.
2. Baker P, Everseley J. *Multi-lingual capital. The languages of London school children and their relevance to economic, social and educational policies.* London: Battlebridge Publications, 2000.
3. Carr-Hill R, Passingham S, Wolf A, Kent N. *Lost opportunities: the language skills of linguistic minorities in England and Wales.* London: Basic Skills Agency, 1996.
4. Ozolins U. *Interpreting and translation in Australia. Current issues and international comparisons.* Melbourne: Language Australia, 1998.
5. Phelan M, Parkman S. How to do it: work with an interpreter. *British Medical Journal* 1995; 311: 555–557.
6. Sanders M. *As good as your word. A guide to community interpreting and translation in public services.* London: The Maternity Alliance, 2000.
7. Levinson R, Gillam S. *Linkworkers in Primary Care.* London: King's Fund, 1998.

Further information

Bradby H. Communication, interpretation and translation. In: Culley L, Dyson S (eds). *Ethnicity and nursing practice.* Basingstoke: Palgrave, 2001.
Jones D, Gill P, Harrison R, *et al.* An exploratory study of language interpretation services provided by video conferencing. *Journal of Telemedicine and Telecare* 2003; 9: 51–56.
Kai J. Cross-cultural communication. *Medicine* 2000; 28(10): 36–38.
Kai J, Briddon D, Bavan J. Working with interpreters and advocates. In: Kai J (ed.). *Valuing Diversity,* 2nd edn. London: Royal College of General Practitioners, 2003.
Sanders M – see reference 6 above – is a very helpful practical resource.

8 Working with link workers and advocates

Akgul Baylav and Jon Fuller

This chapter concerns a group of people providing an important link between health professionals and patients who encounter barriers in accessing health care. Many are employed, paid or unpaid, to work with minority ethnic communities. They have a number of different titles, 'link workers' and 'bilingual health advocates' being perhaps the commonest.

Historically, the concept of having someone to act as the patient's advocate began in the USA in the 1950s and 1960s for people with disabilities, learning difficulties and mental ill health. This idea gradually assumed a place in the UK.

Bilingual advocacy

One of the first initiatives in the UK area was the Hackney Multi-ethnic Women's Health Project, set up in 1980 by the City and Hackney Community Health Council. A team of community workers acted as patient advocates for women from minority ethnic communities using the local maternity services.

This was followed by national initiatives such as the Asian Mother and Baby Campaign in 1982. This attempted to address concerns similar to those in Hackney – the poor outcome of pregnancies among some South Asian communities. In 1990, bilingual health advocacy was transferred to primary care settings spreading from East London to elsewhere in the country.

Principles of advocacy

The principles of advocacy within health care are similar to those of advocates in legal settings – basically, advocates are there to represent the patient's interests to the health service.

The key principles of an advocacy service are that it should be a user or patient-led service; non-judgemental; confidential; independently set up and managed from health service providers and accountable to users and their communities.

It is important that advocates should be employed independently of the health services organizations with which they work. This gives them the freedom to comment without fear of victimization and potential employment problems. Their employer should provide supervision and support, help them keep a sense of perspective and negotiate for them with the health care organization and the community within which they work.

Bilingual advocacy and interpreting

Bilingual link workers, advocates, interpreters, community interpreters and translators are all titles that may be used interchangeably for bilingual workers who are employed to help overcome 'language and cultural barriers'.

However, there can be substantial differences in the ways they operate and in the way issues are addressed. As with most innovations, these differences are not always understood by either patients or providers of health services. They remain subject of ongoing debate (see 'Further information'). Consider the example in Box 8.1.

The roles of an advocate

Advocates carry out their role in a number of ways:

- by educating health care staff about patients' culture and background, socio-economic conditions and the health care needs of their communities
- by supporting patients within consultations by interpreting and explaining what is taking place
- by assisting patient's understanding of why procedures are taking place or the need for particular treatments
- by informing patients about possible choices for the management of their condition, encouraging patients to ask questions
- by ensuring that the patient's needs and concerns are dealt with
- by informing patients about their rights within the system and its institutions
- by challenging practices within the system which discriminate against their client group, by challenging institutional racism or, indeed, racist attitudes and practices by individuals
- by helping to change and improve services and systems by providing consistent and open feedback from patients and their communities to health providers.

One example is the bilingual health advocacy service in East London. The boroughs of Hackney, Tower Hamlets and Newham attempt to provide

Box 8.1 **Comparison of interpreting, link worker and advocacy roles**

Imagine a situation where a patient is unwell and goes to see a doctor. The patient is ill, and feels fragile and vulnerable. She is not familiar with the system and surroundings, speaks little or no English and needs treatment and care. The doctor, from whatever ethnic background, is in her own surroundings, and is knowledgeable and powerful.

Without language support, these two parties cannot speak to each other. They may attempt to communicate with gestures and signs, but this, even with the best of intentions, is prone to misunderstanding and frustration.

Bring into this situation an interpreter. The two parties can at least talk to each other. But this does not necessarily mean they can understand each other. If the patient knows what she needs and is articulate and confident enough to express those needs, then a good interpreter may facilitate effective access to appropriate care for this patient.

Clearly the health professional needs to be willing to explore and address the patient's needs sensitively. Unfortunately a gap in understanding often remains.

A bilingual link worker introduced into this situation will interpret for the patient, their carers and the health professionals involved. He or she will also help shed some light on relevant cultural issues, both in general and specifically for the individual patient. This can work assuming a culturally sensitive and non-discriminatory service.

Unfortunately interpreters and link workers often work to a prescribed brief and may not be permitted to 'interfere' (e.g. go beyond neutral interpretation of language only), even when they experience or observe discrimination towards their clients or communities.

A bilingual advocate may in this case be best placed to negotiate on behalf of, but in partnership with, their clients, and challenge discrimination if and when needed.

Advocates can act independently of health service professionals and providers. They are accountable, first and foremost, to their clients and communities. They attempt to bring health professionals and their patients to an equal level where the available options and outcomes of care for the patient can be freely negotiated (see roles of an advocate below).

comprehensive, though over-stretched, support to facilitate access to health services by minority ethnic communities:

♦ All NHS hospital Trusts employ a number of bilingual health advocates.

♦ A telephone interpreting service is available when face-to-face advocacy is not on hand.

♦ Primary Care Trusts (PCTs) employ teams of advocates to cover the main minority ethnic groups, available for consultations for primary care professionals and community nurses.

♦ To support smaller minority communities, the PCTs have identified a budget for bringing in 'sessional' advocates.

◆ There are also community-based, independent advocacy providers such as DERMAN (providing health advocacy and counselling services for the Turkish and Kurdish communities) in Hackney, Disability Advocacy Network (DAN) in Tower Hamlets or Somali Health Advocacy Project (SHAP) in Newham. They are funded from different sources for the different elements of their work.

Models of working

As local conditions vary, there is no single model applicable to all settings. The main models of providing advocacy services within health care are:

Locally based services

Personal, face-to-face advocacy services are best provided from a local site (e.g. hospital, health centre or a local office or site including community centres and mosques). The advantages are familiarity with the local health service as well as local communities and agencies. This can help accessibility and availability, appropriate referrals to local networks for additional support, on-call during office hours, and outreach/support at home when needed.

Sessional services

These are usually weekly sessions where advocacy is provided on a regular basis from one service site (e.g. maternity, mental health, GP or dental services) for a specific group of patients.

This can help the service provider to focus on the needs of one specific group and arrange other relevant help as necessary (e.g. bilingual receptionists or showing relevant videos in the waiting area). Consistency and predictability of advocacy support increases the uptake of the service. However, this model may mean that patients have to wait for or attempt to fit their 'illnesses' into specific times.

The health educator role

Health advocates can also act to provide patients with education about health and illness, collect health promotion materials relevant to their communities and distribute them, and become involved in health promotion. In some places they have been trained to act independently to obtain information from patients, for instance seeing a pregnant woman before their midwife at booking and taking an antenatal booking history.

Health promotion sessions for groups from the same community with similar ideas, lifestyles and concerns will not only furnish them with much needed information but also with the opportunity to provide mutual support in the community long after the session is over.

Specialist services

Advocates are based within the service (e.g. maternity, cardiology, TB or diabetes clinics) and work only with the users and providers of that specialist service. This gives them a good working knowledge of specialist terminology and familiarity with the services, helps to establish trust between themselves and users (both community members and providers of health services), and continuity of service. Health management, counselling, and support functions may also be integrated (e.g. for maternity, HIV/AIDS or haemoglobinopathies).

Box 8.2 gives an example of advocacy in practice in primary care.

Box 8.2 **Example of advocacy in primary care: 'DERMAN', a non-statutory community based advocacy service in Hackney**

Advocates have timetabled sessions at GP surgeries where they may be working with any of the primary care team members. A half-day session might include a baby clinic and a GP session. Patients are booked in for both health visitor/doctor and advocate, although the community know that the advocate will be on the premises during this session, and patients come along to ask for assistance or with urgent problems.

The organization also answers questions about administrative problems, such as hospital appointments, over the telephone. They have obtained funding for specialist workers, and now have a team of counsellors, a smoking cessation adviser, a parenting worker and a benefits adviser.

Although under-resourced, it appears to be a good model for an advocacy service: it is independent, it is flexible enough to respond to community needs where it can obtain funding, and it can negotiate with GP surgeries and other primary care services about the best way the needs of the Turkish and Kurdish communities can be addressed.

Local GP perspective – working with Turkish/Kurdish patients

'We have struggled over the years to find the best way to provide GP services to our large number of Turkish and Kurdish patients. We have tried no appointment walk-in surgeries, appointment-only surgeries, all doctors seeing Turkish and Kurdish patients during a session, one doctor dedicated to these patients during a session.

We have been helped by feedback from the advocates, their own experiences elsewhere, how it feels doing the work and feedback from patients. The service is not perfect. There are never enough appointments with the advocate, continuity is still a problem and we have to use the telephone interpreting service for patients who turn up as an emergency.

The advocate often becomes trapped across the reception desk dealing with other problems, such as housing. Given the resources, we think we have made the best arrangements we can.'

Working with advocates

Principles for improving the interpreted consultation are discussed in Chapter 7. Facilitation of advocacy is promoted by a number of other factors.

♦ Advocates work best with individual patients by spending time with them before the health consultation to identify and discuss their concerns, and again afterwards to confirm what has happened and make sure the patient is happy and understands advice and instructions fully.

♦ Advocates work best with organizations if time is put aside to develop the relationship between the advocate and clinical and administrative staff. The potential for misunderstanding and distrust is high (see below). This can be ameliorated by improving communication and learning about each other.

♦ Health professionals should expect consultations to take twice as long as un-interpreted consultations. This is the time it takes to convey information three ways. However, one effective consultation saves several consultations that are repeatedly ineffective.

Challenges of working with advocates

There are a number of obvious challenges for health care staff, for advocates and for health service institutions.

Advocate – health professional relationship

Health care staff may find it very difficult to consult with patients in the presence of someone who is essentially a critical observer of what they are doing, and whose job is to encourage the patient to be more assertive.

This is particularly so when the advocate advises a patient that they have the right to consider alternative management options or to ask challenging questions. The higher the stakes in the intervention, the more likely there is to be friction (e.g. where advocates encourage patients to consider alternative care options to obstetricians on labour wards).

Challenging attitudes

Health care staff and institutions can feel defensive when institutional racism is discussed. Staff may resent having to change the way they do things to accommodate a particular minority ethnic community, particularly if they have not been involved in planning a service. They may perceive they are being accused of racism.

Challenges for advocates

Advocates themselves can find their role difficult and challenging. They may need help and support to deal with sensitive issues. Advocates often form good relationships with health care teams and may find it difficult to challenge 'accepted' behaviour.

Collusion can develop between advocate and health professional, which may even progress to blaming the problems encountered on the minority ethnic community rather than considering alternative ways of organizing health care.

Where organizations and individuals have to be challenged, this is a source of emotional stress for the advocate, which can lead to poor morale and high staff turnover in those employed for this role if not adequately supported.

Confidentiality can be a difficult and complex issue, creating conflict or stress. The community with which the advocate works may not always understand and accept the professional role the advocate assumes during their work and may have considerable anxiety about confidentiality, particularly if the community is relatively small and the advocate is drawn from within that community, as they often are.

Advocates must comply with health professional codes of confidentiality. This includes, for example, being requested not to pass on information that a patient may have an unconfirmed malignancy. In addition patients may give advocates information that they ask not to be passed on. For example:

> I am aware of a number of patients who no longer live within (the GP's) catchment area. They have told me not to tell their doctor as they will be asked to find a new GP. They said that there are no advocates who can help them in this (new) area so they want to come here.
> [Bilingual health advocate]

Expectations and demands on advocates

All parties that work with advocates can have high expectations that may not be fulfilled. For some patients, this may be their main contact with English-speaking authority and their best source of bilingual help. They may ask and expect advocates to assist in matters for which the advocate is neither employed nor experienced, such as immigration problems and housing.

Patients may expect the advocate to negotiate with the health service to change the system in a way that is not possible. The community may expect the advocate to institute widespread reforms within a sector of the health service which may be unachievable.

Health professionals, too, may have unrealistic expectations. For instance, advocates cannot be expected to provide counselling unless they have been trained to do so. Similarly, they are not diagnostic assistants to health professionals (e.g. 'I think Mrs X may be severely depressed, what do you think?')

In particular, health professionals cannot expect advocates to effect profound changes in a community's behaviour with respect to health services. There can be a temptation to heap all the frustration of providing health care for a community that does not follow the accepted pattern of behaviour on to the advocate.

Conclusion

Advocacy that acts on behalf of and in partnership with patients to improve their health care presents numerous challenges: at individual and organizational levels, both philosophically and administratively. However, where quality of health care is variable, advocacy has a very important role. For health professionals the presence of an advocate not only facilitates communication with patients, but also provides assistance with the challenges and potential conflicts that diversity may bring.

Key points

- Bilingual advocates primarily represent the interests of the patient and are best employed independently from the organizations with whom they work
- Advocates have a wider role than interpreters, which includes informing patients about their rights, giving feedback on how health systems are working and addressing discriminatory practice
- Health professionals can find the presence of advocates difficult and challenging
- Advocates can find their roles difficult and challenging, and require adequate support
- Both health professionals and patients may have unrealistic expectations of advocates
- Advocates should be welcomed as equal partners with health professionals

Further information

A standards framework for delivering effective health and social care advocacy for black and minority ethnic Londoners. London: King's Fund, 2002.

Baxter C, Baylav A, Fuller J, Marr A, Sanders M. *The case for provision of bilingual services within the NHS.* London: Department of Health, 1996.

Baylav, A. Advocacy in primary health care. In: *Share,* Issue 9. London: Kings Fund, 1994.

Cornwall J, Gordan P. *An experiment in advocacy. The Hackney multi ethnic health project.* London: King's Fund, 1984.

Levenson R. *Linkworkers in primary care.* London: Kings Fund, 1998.

Silvera M, Kapasi, R. *Health advocacy for minority ethnic Londoners.* London: King's Fund, 2000.

9 Health promotion and screening

Lai Fong Chiu

There is a lack of knowledge and understanding among professionals about health promotion and screening in relation to ethnically diverse communities. This has led to a focus on language and culture as the only barriers to health care. For example, in cervical and breast cancer screening these assumptions have led to many professionals regarding 'deficiencies' in minority ethnic women's knowledge, beliefs and attitudes as reasons for non-attendance. Other factors such as the possibility that women's experience of, and satisfaction with the service might affect uptake, are ignored. In addition, the failure to recognize other structural barriers that might affect women's access to health services has perpetuated ineffective health promotion practice.

In the Ottawa Charter for Health Promotion (1986), the World Health Organization called for health promotion – 'Health for All 2000' – through empowerment, advocacy, community participation and organizational change.[1] This formed the philosophical basis of health promotion practice throughout the 1990s. However, the dominance of evidence from randomized controlled trials that can be inappropriately applied to the complex psycho-social aspects of health promotion and screening has limited the development of appropriate evidence to inform effective practice.

This chapter underlines the principles and practice of health promotion by describing the 'Community Health Educator' (CHE) model for cancer screening services. This illustrates key issues, which need to be considered by professionals wishing to adopt effective health promotion programmes for black and minority ethnic (BME) communities.

Principles and practice of health promotion

The Alma Ata declaration (see above) marked a shift in how health professionals conceptualize health, the determinants of health, and the strategies for achieving health. The core principles of health promotion are community participation and empowerment.

However, the lack of a clear understanding of the prerequisites for effective health promotion has led to most health promotion activities (e.g. promoting n, mental or sexual health, cancer screening and the prevention ⎪dedly continuing to encourage individuals to change their ⎪h information-giving alone. To rethink how best to deliver ⎪o a diverse community, the principles and practice set out in ⎪...⎯ of this chapter should be understood and implemented.

Empowerment and community participation

Designing health promotion initiatives to serve communities and not just individuals is at the heart of the new health promotion movement. If we are to accept broader concepts of health, we need to understand the social, political and economic determinants that affect people's health and health behaviours. Underlying the principles of empowerment and community participation is acknowledgement of the inequality of health experienced by disadvantaged and vulnerable groups in our society, and the imbalance of power relationships between health professionals and members of the communities. Practice based on the empowerment principle means that health professionals are willing to share power with communities to enable them to set and achieve their own health agendas.

Community participation assumes that communities are not homogeneous. To meet the diverse health needs of communities, health professionals are required to involve communities. This means seeking equal partnership to participate not only in defining community health agendas, but also in the planning and delivery of health promotion activities in communities. The process of community capacity building is central to the implementation of community participation (see below).

The new health promotion practice

The following are important principles in practising health promotion.

Involving communities to identify needs

Those who are responsible for delivering health promotion programmes need to involve communities in identifying their own health priorities. This means making links between the wider social determinants of health as perceived by local communities and health outcomes defined by the government. For example, the promotion of heart health and cancer prevention will require communities to recognize that heart disease and cancers are serious health problems and to define for themselves the conditions under which changes to promote health are possible.

Developing health promotion solutions with communities

The effective development of health promotion strategies and intervention programmes in a diverse community requires intimate understanding of local conditions. Often, solutions emerge in the process of defining the problems. This process is not only practical and effective, but also facilitates ownership of the interventions by the communities.

Involving stakeholders in programmes

Effective planning and implementation of interventions requires intimate local knowledge and adequate financial and human resources. Greater participation in this process, not only by communities but also local health service and other stakeholders, will increase the likelihood of appropriate and flexible use of health promotion resources. Good local knowledge contributed by communities will enhance coordination.

Involving communities in monitoring and evaluation

Deciding whether an intervention is successful or not requires communities to participate in its assessment. The underlying assumption of participatory monitoring and evaluation is the commitment to a 'learning cycle'. Rather than seeing health outcomes as the only product of health interventions, lessons learnt from an intervention are invaluable for the improvement of future interventions. Involving communities in monitoring and evaluation has the effect of building capacity and community competence.[2]

Effective practice implies not only attention to ways in which health promotion activities are organized, but also the building of health promotion leadership and capacity in primary care.

The following description of the 'Community Health Educator' model highlights the challenges and opportunities for health promotion in diverse communities based on these principles. Other aspects of health promotion relevant to a range of specific clinical areas are considered in Section III of this book.

The Community Health Educator model

The CHE model has been developed through participatory action research to address low uptake of cervical and breast cancer screening among minority ethnic women. It holds community participation and empowerment as central principles.

The concept is based on the recruitment and training of lay members of local communities to deliver health promotion as 'Community Health Educators' (CHEs). Users of screening services are systematically involved through CHEs in the planning and delivery of health promotion programmes with three stages (Figure 9.1).

These three stages embrace the key steps of health promotion practice outlined earlier, involving both professionals and communities throughout the process.

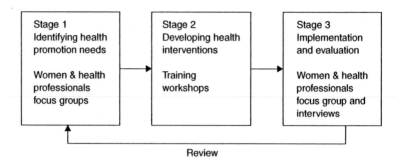

Figure 9.1 The community health educator model in cancer screening

The considerable benefits of involving communities in health promotion initiatives include:

♦ improving the quality and acceptability of services: apart from increasing uptake rates among non-attenders, women ask to access other services such as family planning and sexual health

♦ development of more appropriate, linguistically and culturally sensitive health promotion resources, such as photo-stories depicting a woman's experience of a cervical screening service

♦ opportunity for lasting relationships to be established between primary care practices and their communities.

Many health districts have adopted the CHE model to encourage uptake of cervical and breast screening among minority ethnic women. However, the CHE model has also been applied to other areas of health promotion such as prevention of heart disease (see Chapter 11), sexual health and access to ante-natal services.

Issues that health professionals might note, should they wish to apply the CHE model for health promotion within their own contexts and clinical areas of interest, are now considered. These are relevant to many communities and should be considered whatever the ethnic group.

Recognizing inequality of access to services

A clear recognition of patterns of inequality experienced by minority ethnic communities is essential for targeting resources to areas of most need. Take the case of promoting cancer screening: although national uptake rates on breast and cervical screening are good, there is a large variation among regions. Lower uptake rates have been found in areas with higher concentrations of minority ethnic population and socio-economically disadvantaged communities. This pattern of uptake suggests inequality of access. However, in the absence of systematic ethnic monitoring in primary care (see Chapter 4), it is difficult to determine the degree of local variation, and wide disparities have been found between different general practices.

It is common to find that inequality of access to breast screening is invisible. Neither the organization responsible nor the process of screening is based in the primary care setting. Involving communities to articulate their health promotion needs can help practices confront problems that are perhaps not well understood.

Importance of patient profiling

Patient profiling and its importance for service development and improving quality of care are discussed in Chapter 4. The current lack of ethnicity data including information about clients' language needs makes a planned and targeted approach to health promotion almost impossible.

CHEs have met this challenge by working closely with practice managers, practice nurses and receptionists to identify minority ethnic women who have not attended screening. Since CHEs are women recruited from the neighbourhood, they are well placed to accurately identify the ethnic origin of women who appear on the 'Did Not Attend' (DNA) list, using a combination of names and local knowledge. This can enable a practice to develop a targeted approach to health interventions and other promotion activities.

Developing community health educators

Experience from existing CHE initiatives underlines that promotion of screening requires not only information giving, but also the acknowledgement of the wider social experience of women and how women perceive health and cope with illness. In a diverse community, there is a myriad of perceptions and coping strategies that are influenced by familial and cultural patterns. CHEs recruited from the communities will be able to work with these diverse perspectives.

The assumption that members of ethnically diverse communities who become bilingual workers have the natural linguistic capacity to translate or interpret everything is unwarranted. In return for the local knowledge offered by the CHEs, health professionals need to share technical knowledge with CHEs so that they can translate technical and biomedical terms. Armed with training in health promotion knowledge and skills, CHEs are equipped to inform, educate, and support women to access various services offered by primary care. A well-supported CHE model can act as a vehicle for wider community involvement in health promotion.

A well-constructed training programme for CHEs should include the following components:

- knowledge about the health problem, for example breast and cervical cancers, and the concept of cancer screening
- attitudes and skills needed by effective community health educators or promoters.

Training manuals for training CHEs are published and available in the NHS.[3]

Building health promotion capacity among health professionals

A focus on language and culture as the only factors leading to poor uptake of screening in minority ethnic populations has underplayed the professionals' role in the clinical encounter. The knowledge, attitudes and skills of professionals working with minority ethnic clients are crucial to enhancing the screening experience of women and promoting regular uptake (see Chapter 10).

The successful adoption of the CHE model requires a fundamental shift in the attitude of professionals, a critical rethinking of their role and a willingness to work hand-in-hand with CHEs to promote screening. Critical education that promotes awareness of the relationship between social inequality and health as well as communication skills training is an essential part of health promotion training (see Chapters 6, 7, 8 and 10)

At present there are a few useful resources for the facilitation of health professional training to respond to ethnic diversity.[4] However, the widespread and routine adoption of relevant training is still needed.

Participatory monitoring and evaluation

The sustainability of the CHE model is important if it is to develop its full potential in facilitating health promotion. Participatory monitoring emphasizes the developmental and nurturing process of the CHEs, so that they can become a living entity with the power to respond to change, and can integrate successfully into the primary care team.

Involving communities in the evaluation process following their involvement in the planning and implementation of health promotion programmes and activities is needed. This will ensure that different perspectives are taken into account. The evaluation process can also be an affirming activity in which communities feel accountable for their own thinking and action, thus contributing to capacity building.

Identifying champions and partners

Finally, the setting up of CHE services in health districts is often championed by enthusiastic individuals, for example practice nurses or health promotion specialists, who not only have the political will to address inequality but also the knowledge and skills to work in partnership with key stakeholders and service personnel to enable change. This involves cross-boundary working and cannot happen without the support of others. Public health and health promotion specialists, general practitioners, and practice nurses need to work together to identify local health promotion strategies and priorities.

Conclusion

This chapter has outlined some of the complex issues involved in promoting participation in health promotion and screening, of which linguistic and cultural barriers form only one dimension. Whatever the focus of health promotion and screening, the challenges and principles for addressing them will be similar. The CHE model offers one practical approach to developing and implementing health promotion in practice by developing partnerships between professionals and lay people, health organizations and communities.

Key points

- ◆ Community participation and empowerment are key principles underlying health promotion
- ◆ Involvement of communities includes the process of identifying needs, developing health interventions, and implementing and evaluating programmes
- ◆ The CHE model, developed from a participatory action research approach, is based on these principles
- ◆ Wider application of the CHE model should consider patient profiling, education and training of health professionals and community health educators, a partnership approach and evaluation for sustainability
- ◆ Adequate resources are needed to build health promotion capacity if the CHE model is to be successfully adopted

References

1. World Health Organization. *Ottawa Charter for health promotion*. Canada: Health & Welfare Canada/Canadian Public Health Association, 1986.
2. Coupal F. Participatory monitoring and evaluation for community-driven projects. *On Track* 1997; 3(3). Available online at *http://www.mosaic-net-intl.ca/ontrack.html*

3. Chiu LF. *Woman-to-Woman*: Cervical Screening Training Pack. Rotherham: Department of Health Promotion, Rotherham Health Authority, 1998.
4. Kai J (ed.). *Valuing diversity*, 2nd edn. London: Royal College of General Practitioners, 2003.

Further information

Chiu LF. Extending the team outwards: building partnerships and teamwork with the communities. In: Baxter C. (ed.). *Managing diversity and inequality in health care*. London: Baillière Tindall/Royal College of Nursing, 2001.
Chiu LF, Heywood P, Jordan J, Mckinney P, Dowel T. Balancing the equation: the significance of professional and lay perceptions in the promotion of cervical screening amongst minority ethnic women. *Critical Public Health*, 1999; 9: 5–22.
Shediac-Rizkallah MC, Bone LR. Planning for the sustainability of community-based health programs: conceptual frameworks and future directions for research, practice and policy. *Health Education Research* 1998; 13: 87–108.
Health Development Agency (HDA) publishes reports, research and other guidance concerning minority ethnic health promotion. These are free and can be downloaded from the HDA website (*http://www.hda-online.org.uk*). Examples include:

Active for life: promoting physical activity with black and minority ethnic groups.
Black and minority ethnic groups and tobacco use in England: a practical resource for health professionals.
Black and minority ethnic groups in England: the second health and lifestyle survey.
Closing the gap: setting local targets to reduce health inequalities.
Effectiveness of interventions to promote healthy eating in people from minority ethnic groups: a review.
Ethnic inequalities in health and smoking behaviour. The role of social capital and social support.
Health-related resources for black and minority groups, 2nd edn.
Improving health through community participation.
Inequalities in health and health promotion: insights from the qualitative research literature.
Participatory approaches in health promotion and planning.

10 Learning to respond to diversity

Joe Kai

Relating to others is more difficult when they appear different from us. In a diverse society we need to be willing to accept the discomfort of unfamiliarity and uncertainty that other's difference may bring. Developing knowledge about local cultural practices and beliefs is useful. However, it is unrealistic for health professionals to know about the myriad of different cultural issues that may arise. Rather they should be sensitized to the importance of diversity and develop generic skills to respond.

These include learning the skills to communicate effectively. Chapter 6 considered principles of cross-cultural communication. Chapters 7 and 8 underline the importance of working with bilingual interpreters, link workers and advocates.

This chapter focuses on other aspects of a generic approach important to any health encounter. These are learning to value cultural diversity and respond to the individual, and becoming sensitized to attitudes to difference. An understanding of stereotyping, prejudice and racism is necessary in order to recognize their impact on health and health care, and to challenge their influence.

'At least she speaks some English'

The example in Box 10.1 may illustrate how some of these issues can arise in practice.

Like Dr Cole, professionals, particularly when pressed for time, may fail to interact caringly. They may fail to recognize the impact of both their own and their patient's background on an interaction. They may stereotype patients, making assumptions about their problem or expectations rather than responding to them as individuals. Professionals may also feel uncomfortable because, even when trying their best, responding to diversity can sometimes be hard.

A range of issues is raised by the dysfunctional consultation in Box 10.1, for example:

- Stereotyping of a South Asian woman with 'psychosomatic' abdominal pain.
- Lack of shared language causing mutual frustration for patient and doctor, and affecting diagnosis and care received.
- Difficulties of access to health care – knowledge of appointment systems and the practicalities of doing so without speaking English.

Box 10.1   **'At least she speaks some English' – a consultation in general practice**

Naseem Iqbal has been added as an 'extra' to the end of Dr Cole's surgery. She has come without an appointment, and speaks Punjabi but little English. The receptionist tells him the patient appears to have abdominal pain. Dr Cole's first reaction is to express sarcastic surprise that this is the problem, but he is relieved the patient speaks some English. He's annoyed he's going to be late starting house calls and as the patient sits down he asks her, rather more abruptly than he meant to, why she didn't make an appointment. But she just looks back at him anxiously. She is only able to explain 'too much pain', pointing to her abdomen. He asks if she has been sick (meaning vomiting) and she seems to understand and nod.

Dr Cole has difficulty ascertaining any further history and he becomes impatient. He tells her she has 'gastroenteritis'. On seeing the patient's blank expression he rings through to reception and tells them to give her a leaflet about minor illness on her way out.

Mrs Iqbal then says 'why hurt when go toilet?'. Dr Cole realizes she means dysuria and that his original diagnosis may be wrong. Frustrated, and slightly embarrassed, he hastily gives her a prescription for antibiotics for a possible urinary infection, indicating the consultation has finished.

At this point Mrs Iqbal asks 'no check me doctor?'. Dr Cole is now more embarrassed he has not examined her, especially given the poor history he obtained. He justifies his decision not to examine her by recalling that South Asian women may be uncomfortable with examination by a male doctor. He responds to her request by suggesting she return with an appointment to see his female partner.

From: Kai et al.[1] Reproduced with permission of *Medical Education*

- ◆ Negotiating culturally sensitive issues and treating people as individuals – the doctor excuses himself from examining the patient despite her implicit permission to do so.

- ◆ Assuming the patient can read a leaflet – she is unlikely to read English and may not be literate in her own language even if that material were available.

- ◆ Discrimination and racism in not following up with appropriate interpreting help.

- ◆ The considerable challenges of such consultations, including the difficult feelings and negative attitudes that may arise in professionals themselves.

Valuing cultural diversity: responding to the individual

Health professionals can learn to value diversity by appreciating how variations in culture may affect health and health care. In a health encounter, differences in ethnicity and language may be obvious. However, the 'iceberg model' shown in Figure 10.1 shows that many other important cultural contexts may not be

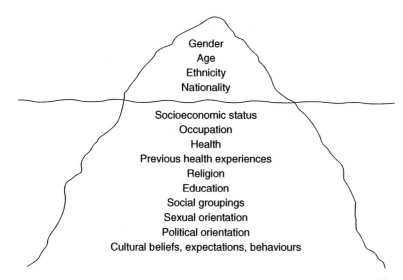

Gender
Age
Ethnicity
Nationality

Socioeconomic status
Occupation
Health
Previous health experiences
Religion
Education
Social groupings
Sexual orientation
Political orientation
Cultural beliefs, expectations, behaviours

Figure 10.1 Iceberg model of cultural influences on health encounters. Reproduced with permission of the Royal College of General Practitioners from Kai J (ed.), *Valuing Diversity – a resource for effective health care of ethnically diverse communities.* London: Royal College of General Practitioners, 1999

readily apparent and may remain unrecognized – below the surface – unless they are considered.

Responding effectively means being sensitive to an individual's culture in its broadest dynamic sense – not only a patient's ethnicity but also their socio-economic background, education, prior health experiences, religion, and so on. Professionals can then contextualize the health and health care experiences of patients as individuals. In particular they need to appreciate the importance of structural influences on health care experience, such as racism and social inequality.

What's your culture?

We all have a culture. Health professionals, just like patients, approach health encounters with their own unique backgrounds, beliefs and ways of communicating. Thus professionals need to be aware of how differences between themselves and their patients may affect their interactions with patients.

Developing cultural self-awareness can be a challenge. We are rarely asked to reflect on who we are. We may also feel vulnerable. Anything that questions the nature of our identity can be threatening. Bearing in mind the iceberg model in Figure 10.1, consider these questions:

♦ What comprises your culture (both that which may be apparent to a stranger, and that which is less obvious about you)?

♦ What makes up your health professional culture (backgrounds, attitudes and behaviours shared with your health professional colleagues)?

♦ How might these affect your communication with patients?

For example, although a GP may share the same ethnicity as his patient, other differences between them such as professional status, power, gender and socio-economic background may shape and potentially compromise their interaction.

Attitudes to difference

Learning effective communication skills, and developing sensitivity to cultural diversity in others and ourselves are key steps. Recognition of our attitudes and prejudices, and society's attitudes towards those who appear different from us are equally important.

Rather than reflect on their attitudes to diversity, health professionals and those in training may often prefer simply to learn about 'ethnic' differences, for example differing dietary, death or bereavement practices.[3] Of course, learning about these aspects of culture in one's local communities can be valuable where feasible (see 'Further information,' below). However, we may all, consciously or unconsciously, hold stereotyped, negative or racist attitudes towards others.

Stereotyping

All of us have a tendency to stereotype – that is to assume people have certain perspectives or characteristics because they appear to belong to a certain group (see Box 10.2). Developing stereotypes seems to be a way that we cope with the uncertainty of the world and attempt to make life more predictable. However, the effects

---

Box 10.2   Some examples of stereotyping from real life

- A practice nurse decides it's not worth discussing weight loss with an African-Caribbean woman with hypertension because she assumes her patient will not be receptive to dieting and a 'Western' ideal of healthy slimness
- A medical student seeing a Bangladeshi man with poorly controlled diabetes notes he is not taking the two different drugs prescribed. He records 'poor compliance' in the records. In fact the patient can only afford one drug prescription charge
- A GP may make assumptions about South Asian consanguineous marriage and congenital malformations in children:
  '...The first thing he asks is, 'Is it a first cousin marriage? You've had one disabled child, then another' He's a good doctor but, because of his attitude, I only go when I really have to. I feel embarrassed or ashamed almost. I feel that they must wonder what kind of system Pakistani people have, or that we don't have any sense'

(A Pakistani Muslim woman caring for a daughter with a physical disability)[4]

of stereotyping are harmful and the process unethical. Avoiding making assumptions and responding to a patient as an individual must be the guiding principle.

Prejudice and discrimination

When stereotyped people become victims of narrow judgements and of prejudice – opinions or views (usually unfavourable) formed without knowledge, thought or reason.

Discrimination occurs when prejudice is acted on so that people are treated unfairly or differently because they belong to a particular group. Health professionals must recognize that prejudice and discrimination exist in health services, and that how they respond to patients can affect patients' experiences of them.

The nature of racism

Racism occurs when an ideology of power and superiority of one ethnic group over another is used to justify discrimination. 'Race', as discussed in Chapter 1, is a problematic concept. Nonetheless racism often refers to oppression based on very superficial physical 'racial' differences such as (typically non-white) skin colour or facial appearance. At the same time, many white minorities such as the Irish, Jewish or Traveller communities experience racism as a result of other cultural differences.

Racism is not easy to define but a working definition usually combines:

◆ a philosophy and practice of ethnic power and superiority that affects the conscious or unconscious behaviour of individuals and society

◆ assumptions, stereotyping and prejudice

◆ discrimination.

At the heart of racism is the lasting impact that historical colonial power and domination have made on how white (and black) people think. This has imbued societies with the notion of white superiority over black people.

There has always been racism. In Shakespeare's *The Merchant of Venice* the Prince of Morocco begins his case for the hand of Portia by apologizing for his colour – 'Mislike me not for my complexion' he pleads, taking it for granted that Portia will be prejudiced. And he is right – she has already declared her distaste: 'if he have the condition of a saint, and the complexion of a devil, I had rather he should shrive me than wive me'.

Centuries later, in today's health service, some people continue to experience the same derogatory treatment. For example:[5]

◆ The doctor put his gloves on to examine me – it was as if I had a contagious disease because I was a refugee and African.

◆ The receptionist said, 'You are too demanding, you get better treatment here than wherever you came from.'

Racism in health care

Racism is a pervasive feature of wider society and public institutions. This includes health services and interactions between professionals and patients.[6,7] These are as much shaped by broader social assumptions and stereotyping as by the existence of direct prejudice.[8] Different and overlapping forms of racism may occur:

♦ *Direct racism*: where a person is treated less favourably simply by virtue of their ethnicity.

♦ *Ethnocentrism*: where inappropriate assumptions are made about the needs of some people on the basis of the ethnic majority experience. For example, that the gender of a health professional is not particularly important to a patient.

♦ *Indirect or institutional racism*: where, although services are apparently provided equally to all people, the form in which they are provided inevitably disadvantages some groups. For example, lack of provision of interpreting, providing information in languages other than English or facilities to pray that are limited to those of Christian faith. Institutional racism has been usefully defined in the landmark Macpherson Report following the racist murder of Stephen Lawrence[9] (see Box 10.3).

Responding to racism: facilitating learning and behaviour

It is difficult to change peoples' attitudes, even if it is felt to be desirable. However, in health care two steps may allow practical progress.

♦ Better training that can inform staff attitudes – at all levels of the NHS.

♦ Achieving clarity about expected responsibilities and standards of behaviour in practice.

Box 10.3 **Definition of institutional racism[9]**

The collective failure of an organization to provide an appropriate and professional service to people because of their colour, culture or ethnic origin. It can be seen or detected in processes, attitudes and behaviour which amount to discrimination through unwitting prejudice, ignorance, thoughtlessness and racist stereotyping which disadvantages ethnic minority people...

[Racism] persists because of the failure of the organization openly and adequately to recognize and address its existence and causes by policy, example and leadership. Without recognition and action to eliminate such racism it can prevail as part of the ethos or culture of the organization. It is a corrosive disease.

Some people will inevitably have more negative attitudes to diversity than others. However, regardless of what attitudes people may hold, it is ultimately people's behaviour that matters. Moreover, appropriate standards of behaviour in practice can be more easily measured and monitored.

Health professional training to respond to diversity

Recent moves to promote equality and diversity training in the NHS, starting at senior board level, are welcome.[10] Modest progress is being made in some health professional curricula where relevant training has been either patchy or non-existent.[1,11,12]

One approach is to encourage reflection on attitudes in ways that can inform them, and promote self-awareness and learning. This offers opportunities to inform an understanding of appropriate behaviour and good practice. The aim is to develop transferable skills that enable a flexible response to diversity.[1,2,11] This means learning to become aware of one's own attitudes and prejudices, being sensitive to racism and stereotyping, and respecting the individuality of all patients. These should be regarded as integral to professionals' routine practice or consultation skills.

Strategies to encourage this sort of reflective practice in the context of skills training (e.g. learning how to work with interpreters) may be more successful than overt attempts to change attitudes.[11] In addition, people with the most open of attitudes still need to develop appropriate skills. A skills-based approach may also be less threatening for most practitioners. People's competencies and behaviour can then be assessed. Reflection on issues raised during skills training (e.g. learning how to develop effective information for health promotion) might also inform attitude change.[11]

Box 10.4 suggests some actions that health professionals and others might take in challenging racism and its influence.

Box 10.4   What can you do about racism?

The combined action of individuals makes a difference.

- Recognize societal racism is unconsciously internalized by us all. This is not your fault
- Do not feel guilty and thus feel paralysed to act. You can do something
- Develop greater awareness of your attitudes to difference and your behaviours
- Participate in and promote appropriate equality and diversity training
- Review your working practices – for example, consider and implement ways of improving quality of care for diverse communities (see overview in Chapter 3)
- Promote steps to achieve a representative workforce and tackle racial harassment of staff and patients (see 'Further reading', below)[10]

It is important not to underestimate the internal discomfort generated within health professionals as they approach issues of diversity and difference. For success, this training needs to become embedded in the education, assessment and accreditation of health workers.[1,11] It will take time to empower health professional teachers, clinicians and others in the NHS to teach these skills[11] and to allow appropriate approaches to develop.[1,2,3,11]

Focus on expected standards of behaviour

As opportunities for professionals' learning grow and shape their frameworks for practice, these must be linked to ways of facilitating and reviewing professional behaviour.

As noted in Chapter 3, clinical governance in the NHS to ensure quality of and accountability for care[13] offers a crucial opportunity to do this. At the same time the new Race Relations Amendment Act (2000) now places a duty on public bodies to go beyond preventing discrimination and take steps to promote race equality.

Clinical governance frameworks can articulate standards for quality of care that include non-discriminatory practice and behaviour reflecting positive and appropriate practice (Box 10.5).

Continuing professional training, audit, and review of patients' experiences of care should underpin implementation and monitoring of quality of care. Such steps would go some way to tackling racism in health care and to ensuring equitable and effective care for diverse communities across the NHS.

Clearly tackling racism, social and health inequality also requires broader political, institutional and social change. However, this should not detract the NHS and practitioners from setting measurable standards, such as those above, and monitoring subsequent actions that are achievable now.

Box 10.5   **Examples of standards of behaviour**

- Progress in adopting patient profiling and use of that information to improve care
- The proportion of health encounters using trained interpreting help where indicated
- Provision of culturally sensitive information when required
- Levels of referral from primary to secondary care for chronic disease (where evidence of inappropriately low referral exists)
- Availability of health professional of preferred gender

Conclusion

Diversity makes working in health care both challenging and stimulating. Practitioners need to develop a willingness to understand each patient's perspective and the influence of his or her culture. Regardless of what little they may 'know' about particular cultures, this means that within health encounters they should learn to be aware of their own attitudes and prejudices, avoid stereotyping and respond to patients as individuals. In doing so they can improve quality of care for patients, and address racism through their behaviour. If health practitioners can learn to respond effectively to diversity, they can apply these principles to the benefit of all patients of whatever background.

Key points

- Learn to communicate effectively
- Health professionals have their own culture that affects interactions with patients
- Avoid stereotyping: respond to patients as individuals
- Become aware of your assumptions and attitudes about others
- Be sensitive to racism and challenge its influence

References

1. Kai J, Spencer J, Wilkes M, Gill P. Learning to value ethnic diversity – what, why and how? *Medical Education* 1999; 33: 616–623.
2. Kai J (ed.). *Valuing diversity, 2nd edition.* London: Royal College of General Practitioners, 2003. This training resource book and video provides guidance, practical suggestions and teaching materials for educators to use or modify in order to facilitate small group interactive learning to respond to diversity in health care. It can be used in the training of pre and post-registration health professionals, including medical students, nurses and primary care practitioners. Themes include valuing cultural diversity, developing effective communication, working with interpreters, and understanding racism.
3. Kai J, Bridgewater R, Spencer J. 'Just think of TB and Asians, that's all I ever hear': medical learners' views about training to work in an ethnically diverse society. *Medical Education* 2001; 35: 250–256.
4. Katbamna S, Bhakta P, Ahmed W, *et al.* Supporting South Asian carers and those they care for: role of the primary health care team. *British Journal of General Practice* 2002; 52: 300–305.
5. Yee L. *Breaking barriers: towards culturally competent general practice.* London: Royal College of General Practitioners, 1997.
6. Ahmad WIU. *'Race' and health in contemporary Britain.* Buckingham: Open University Press, 1993.

7. Bowler I. 'They're not the same as us': midwives' stereotypes of South Asian descent maternity patients. *Sociology of Health and Illness* 1993; 15: 157–178.

8. Smaje C. *Health, 'race' and ethnicity, making sense of the evidence.* London: King's Fund, 1995.

9. MacPherson W. *The Stephen Lawrence inquiry.* Report of an inquiry by Sir William Macpherson of Cluny. London: The Stationery Office, 1999.

10. *Promoting equality and diversity in the NHS.* A concise guide developed by the Department of Health including recent changes in equality legislation, important sources of information and recommendations on good employment and workforce practice, and a check list for NHS organizations in making progress on diversity. Although targeted at NHS Board members it is useful for others working in health care. Available online at *http://www.doh.gov.uk/equality/index.htm.*

11. Kai J, Spencer J, Woodward N. Wrestling with ethnic diversity: toward empowering educators. *Medical Education* 2001; 35: 262–271.

12. Gerrish K, Husband C, Mackenzie J. *Nursing for a multi-ethnic society.* Buckingham: Open University Press, 1996.

13. NHS Executive. *Clinical governance. Quality in the new NHS.* London: Department of Health, 1999.

Further information

There are several texts considering aspects of cultural diversity in relation to health. Examples include:

Karmi G (ed.). *The ethnic health handbook: a fact file for health care professionals.* Oxford: Blackwell Science, 1996. This handbook provides practical facts relevant to health care on over twenty ethnic groups and their different religions. This includes, for example, coverage of naming systems and titles; religious festivals, obligations and practices; diet; social customs; cultural issues concerning birth and death; and other specific health issues. The book also lists relevant national and local contacts.

Sheikh A, Gatrad AR (eds.). *Caring for Muslim patients.* Abingdon: Radcliffe, 2000. This book seeks to promote better-informed dialogue about the interface between faith and health. It profiles the Islamic worldview and its concepts of health and disease. Muslim practices and customs of relevance to health and health care are explored and illustrated.

Helman C. *Culture, health and illness,* 4th edn. London: Arnold, 2001. This provides a perspective on medical anthropology applied in a clinical context.

The King's Fund (*http://www.kingsfund.org.uk*) has a range of free downloadable reports and articles concerning minority ethnic health, in addition to relevant publications available from its bookshop. Examples include *Racism in medicine: an agenda for change,* edited by Naz Coker (2001).

Section III
Clinical care in practice

11 Coronary heart disease

Azhar Farooqi and Kamlesh Khunti

Coronary heart disease (CHD) is a major cause of morbidity and mortality in the UK. Its prevention and treatment are a high priority for the NHS, not least because of the high social and economic costs of premature death and illness. CHD is largely a disease of a 'western' type of lifestyle. The impact of the disease on some minority populations, in particular South Asian communities, might be regarded a salutary lesson on how social environments affect health. This chapter highlights the importance of effective primary and secondary prevention of CHD, alongside ways of improving access to health services for minority communities.

Coronary heart disease among ethnic minorities

Higher rates of CHD among South Asians have been noted since the early 1970s, and have been confirmed in a number of studies.[1] Mortality from CHD is 38% higher in South Asian men and 43% higher in South Asian women than in their European counterparts[2] (see Table 11.1).

These findings are replicated in South Asian origin communities living western lifestyles around the world, including urban centres in the Indian sub-continent.

Table 11.1 Mortality from coronary heart disease in South Asians. Relative risk compared to national average (SMR = 1 for England and Wales)

	Men	Women
Brent (Gujarati)	1.6	1.6
Ealing (Punjabi)	1.5	2.1
Tower Hamlets (Bangladeshi)	1.4	
Waltham Forest (Pakistani)	1.6	
1991 Census data	1.38	1.43

The causes of this 'epidemic of CHD' among South Asians are incompletely understood though being explored (for further discussion, see Bhopal[1]).

Of particular note in British data are seemingly higher rates for CHD among South Asian women (Table 11.1)[2] and the markedly higher risk in younger age groups. Compared to a relative risk of 1.38 for those aged 20–69, the relative risks are even higher for South Asian younger men (3.1 for those aged 20–29, and 2.1 for men aged 30–39), compared to those of European origin. There is also evidence that the severity of CHD may be greater in South Asians, with the 6-month mortality for South Asians after a myocardial infarction (MI) reported to be twice that of Europeans.[3] These statistics have significant implications for health care planning, particularly for the urban areas of the UK where there is a young and growing South Asian population.[4]

Although South Asian communities are diverse, they all seem to share increased risk. There are no significant differences between South Asians from Pakistan, Bangladesh and from different regions of India (e.g. Sikhs from the Punjab and Hindus from Gujarat province) in terms of burden of disease. Although differences due to different socio-economic experience may emerge with time.

There is no evidence that African-Caribbean populations of the UK have higher rates of CHD than Europeans. Indeed, despite their high prevalence of hypertension and stroke (see Chapter 13), mortality from CHD appears to be lower in these communities. However, it should be noted that data from the USA shows that falling CHD rates in white populations have not been mirrored in black communities with the consequence that mortality between the two groups is now almost equivalent.

Primary prevention of CHD in South Asians

Primary prevention can be effective in reducing mortality and morbidity from CHD. In deciding on appropriate interventions for South Asians, it is worth exploring the role of different risk factors for CHD among this group. CHD risk scores calculated from risk tables (e.g. the Sheffield table) are based on data derived from a white community. It is generally accepted that such tables underestimate cardiac risk for South Asians.

However, the potential risk factors for South Asians are common to other populations. They include diet and cholesterol, obesity, smoking, physical inactivity, hypertension, alcohol and stress. In addition, the role of diabetes and insulin resistance may be particularly significant for South Asians.

Diet and cholesterol

The evidence suggests that diets of the various South Asian groups may in some respects be healthier than the diet of Britons of European origin. One study suggested that energy from both saturated and total fat is slightly lower among South Asians, particularly vegetarian groups, compared to the general population.

Limited evidence seems to show that plasma cholesterol levels are generally lower among South Asians compared to native Britons. However, cholesterol and fat intake is significantly higher in British Asians compared to Asians in the sub-continent. This raises the issue of what are 'normal' or acceptable lipid levels for different ethnic groups.

Obesity

Comparison of body mass index (BMI) in British South Asians and their European counterparts have shown similar BMIs between men, but South Asian women tend to have a slightly higher index than their European counterparts. Exceptions to this include Bangladeshi men and women who tend to have lower BMIs. The fact that British South Asians have significantly higher BMIs compared to South Asians in the sub-continent again raises the question of what is an ethnically acceptable range.

There is evidence of a different distribution of body fat, with central obesity being more common among South Asians. This is associated with specific metabolic changes, which may result in the development of CHD. Primary care based programmes for the control of obesity in South Asians should include individuals with a BMI of 27–30 (in addition to those with the 'conventional' obesity level of >30), and should also include those with central obesity (waist/hip ratio >1).

Smoking

Smoking is a key risk factor for developing CHD. Smoking practice among South Asians is variable, perhaps reflecting religious and cultural influences. Hindu and Pakistani men seem to have levels of smoking close to the national average, whereas Sikh men and South Asian women in general have lower levels of smoking. However, Bangladeshi men have much higher rates of smoking than other populations.

Physical activity

A number of studies have reported lower leisure-time physical activity in both South Asian men and women compared to non-South Asians. Higher unemployment levels in South Asian men and particularly women, resulting in reduced non-leisure physical activity, probably compound this.

Hypertension

Hypertension is a risk factor for CHD. There is no firm data to suggest prevalence is greater among South Asian groups than Europeans. However, comparison between ethnic groups is difficult when the physiologically optimum levels are not accurately defined.

Diabetes and insulin resistance

There is a strong correlation between type 2 diabetes and CHD. The prevalence of type 2 diabetes is much higher among South Asians than among Europeans, with studies showing prevalence of 20% for South Asians aged 40–65, and over 30% for South Asians over 65 (see Chapter 12).

Although most South Asians with CHD do not have overt diabetes, they often have raised insulin levels. This phenomenon of 'insulin resistance' is associated with the development of central obesity, hypertriglyceridaemia and increased CHD risk. The tendency to insulin resistance is also apparent in South Asian children, in whom it may reflect an increased tendency to adiposity.

Alcohol

The influence of alcohol intake on CHD demonstrates a U-shaped curve, with low/moderate alcohol consumption seeming to confer some protection. Many Asian groups (in particular Muslims) drink little or no alcohol. Some groups (e.g. Sikhs) appear to have a high alcohol intake, particularly amongst men.[1]

Stress

'Stress' as a concept is difficult to define but can be related to loss of control over life events. Whether and how 'stress' may be related to CHD is controversial. It is known that CHD as a totality cannot be completely accounted for by established risk factors. Furthermore, the prevalence of CHD is higher among deprived populations who experience socio-economic stress. Some proven risk factors (e.g. hypertension and smoking) also have an association with stress. It is a reasonable hypothesis that immigrant status, socio-economic deprivation, cultural changes, and racism experienced by South Asians lead to higher stress levels.

Promoting primary prevention among South Asians

From the description of the potential risk factors above it is clear that there is significant scope for primary prevention among South Asians. Many of the issues that need to be addressed by primary prevention are common to all communities. This includes advice and intervention related to smoking, cholesterol, hypertension, diet and exercise. Given evidence of reduced physical activity among South Asians, and the metabolic consequences of insulin resistance, physical activity and dietary advice with the reduction of obesity appear particularly important.

Reports of increased insulin resistance in young South Asians mean that the prevention of obesity in childhood and adolescence, with a combination of dietary measures and increased physical activity, are a strong priority to reduce diabetes and CHD in later life. This provides challenges for schools, communities and services in partnership working.

Physical activity

Increased levels of physical activity assist weight reduction, cardiovascular fitness and reduction in insulin resistance. Issues for health promotion include education and raising awareness for the need for exercise. This includes prompting a more active lifestyle (e.g. the encouragement of walking) as well as increased formal exercise (e.g. via sport and use of leisure centres).

Barriers to improving levels of physical activity

These include factors common to all, such as time and motivation. There is also evidence that there may be lack of awareness among older South Asians of the value of exercise, as well as specific cultural barriers to a more active lifestyle. Examples of this include lack of appropriate facilities for women and older people, for example single-sex exercise facilities and access to exercise in community centres. Financial barriers for some poor income groups may be a deterrent, for example in using leisure centres.

Promoting physical activity

In order to have a significant chance of impact, health promoters need to effectively communicate the value of exercise. This includes the use of mass media (e.g. Asian radio stations) and the more effective use of established community organizations (e.g. women's and religious groups). A number of innovative projects have now begun to address this issue creatively and in ways that enhance their cultural appropriateness. These are varied, promoting for example community walking activities (e.g. the British Heart Foundation 'Chalo Chaleey' project in Leicester), women's gardening groups, and Asian dance as exercise.

Health professionals can have some impact, for example by using 'exercise on prescription' schemes (where a GP, for example, prescribes exercise sessions at a local leisure centre). However, there is no doubt that any significant increase in physical activity must be related to local community action. This principle of effective health promotion is emphasized in Chapter 9. South Asian people need to be empowered with the knowledge and the opportunity to increase levels of activity within their established community structures.

Dietary and smoking advice

Impact on diet is likely to be achieved by education and empowerment of the individual. This includes providing information on risk, and healthy eating advice that is culturally sensitive. The latter is important – to be effective, suggestions have to be practical within a normal Asian diet.

Specific cooking advice, which reduces fat content, but maintains use of basic ingredients and traditional taste, is important. Again the use of media (radio, television) and community groups is a feasible mechanism for large-scale education. Health care professionals themselves need to be equipped with knowledge and appropriate materials to support this process in the context of the advice they give. The British Heart Foundation, for example, have a produced an excellent 'healthy' cookbook for South Asians. Professionals may need specific training to ensure they can fulfil this education role effectively.

An example of community action with respect to diet includes working with Indian restaurants to provide low-fat alternatives on their menus. This is timely – as some South Asians become more prosperous, they are increasingly dining out.

Specific initiatives to tackle high smoking in some South Asian groups include the British Heart Foundation Asian Quitline (see 'Further information'), and the Project Dil Asian smoking cessation clinic in Leicester funded by a local Health Action Zone. This involves a trained, multilingual South Asian smoking cessation counsellor working with local communities.

Knowledge and attitudes to risk factors

For prevention to be effective it needs to be culturally sensitive, accessible and relevant for the target population. There has been limited research exploring the knowledge and attitudes of South Asians to risk factors for heart disease. This seems to indicate that South Asians have a diversity of attitudes and practices with respect to risk factors. Older individuals and non-English-speakers tend to have poorer knowledge about diet, exercise, smoking and alcohol, whereas younger English-speaking South Asians tend to be more aware of these issues.[6]

Health care professionals need to take account of this variation; in particular, it is important not to stereotype South Asians with respect to their knowledge base. Health promotion advice needs to be personally tailored, and good practice should involve identifying the needs of individual patients taking account of their existing understanding and perspective.

Qualitative studies have also shown that even when patients are aware of issues related to risk there are often culturally specific barriers in addressing these. Health care professionals need to be aware of this when giving advice. For example, it may be inappropriate to refer a Muslim woman to swimming classes or a leisure centre without women-only facilities.

Access to health care services

General considerations for access to services are discussed in Chapters 3 and 5. Provision of good-quality health promotion requires organization, accessibility and resources. Often primary care in inner city areas of greatest need (where many minority ethnic communities are concentrated) is the least well resourced, for example in terms of premises and staff.

Inner city practices are more likely to offer 'open' access surgeries rather than booked appointments. This is often a pragmatic response to high acute work-load in disadvantaged communities that may enhance access for patients (e.g. families with ill young children or patients with acute and multiple social issues). However, a relative lack of longer, planned consultations with time to focus on prevention of disease may compromise the quality and quantity of health promotion activity.

Language is a barrier for some South Asians accessing health services. It is self-evident that a nurse or doctor who cannot directly communicate with the patient will find providing effective health promotion problematic. This can potentially be overcome (at least partly) with investment in longer consultations, appropriate health promotion materials and effective interpretation services (see Chapters 3, 6, 7, 8). Specific clinics for health promotion activity can also help to facilitate this.

A practical example of poorly organized health promotion is the common failure to offer screening and advice to first-degree relatives of South Asian patients who have had a myocardial infarction (this sub-group having a 10-fold risk of CHD).

Training in clinical issues related to ethnic minorities, and cultural awareness for health care professionals, are important in helping to address some these issues (see Chapter 10). Undeniably services in deprived areas require greater resources, but an important issue is to develop primary health care teams as effective organizations able to maximize the resources they have.

An example of an innovative approach to primary prevention is Project Dil[7] in Leicester. Box 11.1 below summarizes the key elements of this successful initiative. Central to the approach is the careful selection and training of lay individuals to deliver culturally specific health promotion messages to their own communities.

Box 11.1 **Project Dil[7] – Reducing risk factors in South Asians in Leicester**

- training of 'peer educators' (nationally accredited course with Open College Network)
- peer education events in community and health centres
- development of translated educational materials
- training of health care professionals in effective CHD health care provision
- peer education for cardiac rehabilitation
- Asian language smoking cessation clinic

Secondary prevention for South Asians with CHD

Secondary prevention of CHD should be implemented in all patients with CHD including South Asians, using similar principles. However, the following points merit particular emphasis for people from South Asian communities.

Reducing mortality after myocardial infarction

Studies have demonstrated higher mortality (two-fold) after MI among South Asians compared to Europeans. This may be related to post-infarction hyperglycaemia. Suggested recommendations include:

- use of higher doses of aspirin (300 mg)
- adequate beta blockade
- tight control of glucose levels
- appropriate investigation for cardiac revascularization
- cardiac revascularization if appropriate.

The causes of the higher mortality South Asians experience may also have other explanations. There is some controversial evidence that South Asians do not receive adequate investigation, with procedures such as coronary revascularization (e.g. coronary angioplasty or bypass surgery) being less common. This is particularly worrying as appropriate investigation (i.e. coronary imaging and angiography) can reveal the presence of coronary vessel disease amenable to surgery. In the light of this, and reported concern about discrimination in the NHS, such differences need to be further explored.

Cardiac rehabilitation

Discrimination is not always overt; it may be institutional. For example the generally low uptake of cardiac rehabilitation services by South Asians may be related to issues of language, accessibility and cultural appropriateness. In Leicester, the use of trained 'peer educators' who discuss rehabilitation with MI patients both on the hospital wards and in patients' homes has helped increase uptake of rehabilitation programmes (see Box 11.1).[6]

Other considerations

Health care professionals should also adopt specific strategies for the secondary prevention of CHD among South Asians,[7,8] including:

- ensuring patients understand their illness using interpretation where appropriate
- avoidance of drugs such as thiazides for hypertension, as these may raise blood glucose levels

- where appropriate, selection of lipid lowering drugs which reduce trigly-cerides as well as cholesterol
- aiming for low fat intake in the diet (reduce fat to 21% of total energy intake)
- screening for diabetes on a regular basis.

Conclusion

Coronary heart disease is a major health issue for all majority and minority ethnic communities, and in particular South Asian communities in the UK. CHD can be prevented and when it occurs there are effective treatments. Although the key approaches to primary and secondary prevention are generic to all populations, South Asians require tailored approaches to ensure that barriers to effective health promotion and ensuring equitable access to health services are addressed.

Key points

- Weight reduction and increasing physical activity, together with reducing smoking in some groups, need special attention (it is no coincidence this also reduces the impact of Type 2 diabetes)
- Health promotion, education and interventions require approaches which take account of the language and culture of South Asians
- Existing cardiac risk calculations/tables underestimate cardiac risk in South Asians
- Poor access by South Asians to primary care and other services needs to be addressed
- Secondary prevention of CHD amongst South Asians, with screening for diabetes, and appropriate cardiac investigation and revascularization, can be improved

References

1. Bhopal R. Epidemic of cardiovascular disease in South Asians. *BMJ* 2002; 324: 625–626. This editorial provides a very useful and brief summary of current evidence on high cardiovascular risk in South Asians.
2. McKeigue P, Marmot M. Mortality from coronary heart disease in Asian communities in London. *BMJ* 1998; 297: 903.
3. Balarajan J. Ethnic difference in mortality from ischaemic heart disease and cerebrovascular disease in England and Wales. *BMJ* 1991; 302: 560–564.
4. Wilkinson P, Sayer J, Koorithottumkal L, *et al*. Comparison of case fatality in South Asians and white patients after acute myocardial infarction: an observational study. *BMJ* 1996; 312: 1330–1333.

5. Lowry A, Woods K, Bosha J. The effects of demographic change on CHD mortality in a large migrant population at risk. *Journal of Public Health Medicine* 1991; 276–280.

6. Farooqi A, Nagra D. Attitudes to lifestyle risk factors for coronary heart disease amongst South Asians: A focus group study. *Family Practice* 2000; 17: 293–296.

7. Farooqi A, Bhavsar M. Project Dil: A co-ordinated primary care and community health promotion programme for reducing risk factors of coronary heart disease amongst the South Asian community of Leicester – experiences and evaluation of the project. *Ethnicity and Health* 2001; 6(3/4): 265–270.

8. Kooner J. Reducing CHD mortality in Indian Asians. *Heart* 1997; 78(6): 530.

Further information

The British Heart Foundation (*http://www.bhf.org.uk*) publishes a range of useful patient information concerning the prevention and management of heart disease, translated into different languages.

Health Development Agency: relevant free information can be downloaded from the HDA website (*http://www.hda-online.org.uk*). Examples of publications include:

Active for life: promoting physical activity with black and minority ethnic groups.

Black and minority ethnic groups and tobacco use in England: a practical resource for health professionals.

Coronary heart disease guidance.

Coronary heart disease: contrasting the health beliefs and behaviours of South Asian communities.

Ethnicity, health and health behaviour: a study of older groups. Summary report of main findings.

Opportunities for and barriers to good nutritional health in minority ethnic groups.

Patient information:

Health-related resources for black and minority groups, 2nd edn.

Looking after your heart (available in Bengali, Gujarati, Hindi and Punjabi).

12 Diabetes

Kamlesh Khunti and Azhar Farooqi

An epidemic of type 2 diabetes is emerging across the developing world, and people from some communities are particularly predisposed. Diabetes can have a major impact on the physical, psychological and material well-being of individuals and their families, and can lead to multisystem complications. Furthermore, the economic burden of diabetes is considerable, with major implications for health care resources and most costs being for complications of diabetes. Even small changes in the delivery or quality of care for people with diabetes may therefore have enormous financial consequences.

Prevalence of type 2 diabetes

Diabetes is more common in people originating from the Indian sub-continent than in those from Europe. For example, in one study the age-adjusted prevalence of type 2 diabetes was 3.2% in European males and 4.7% in females compared to 12.4% and 11.2% in South Asian males and females respectively.[1] The prevalence of impaired glucose tolerance was also higher in South Asians aged below 60 years. Furthermore, diabetes remains undiagnosed in up to 40% of South Asians.[1] These findings have been replicated in other research. The age at presentation of diabetes is earlier in South Asians and since duration of diabetes is a strong risk factor for complications this group is at high risk. Diabetes also appears much commoner in African-Caribbean communities than in the population as a whole. One early study found that the prevalence of diabetes among the West Indian community was nearly double that of the indigenous UK white population.[2] In Chinese people the prevalence appears on a par with the white population, but they appear to have higher prevalence of impaired glucose tolerance suggesting a rise in diabetes may be imminent.

Cardiovascular complications of diabetes

Mortality from heart disease is approximately three times higher in South Asian patients with diabetes compared to those with diabetes born in England and

Wales.[3] Furthermore, South Asians with type 2 diabetes are more likely to develop premature coronary heart disease than their white British counterparts. Studies examining mortality rates and complications in people of African-Caribbean origin are limited. One study showed that mortality from stroke in African-Caribbeans with diabetes is nearly four times higher than that of the general population in England and Wales.[3] However, coronary heart disease deaths in African-Caribbean born men with diabetes are not significantly higher than those of people born in England and Wales.

Insulin resistance, which is commonly associated with obesity, type 2 diabetes, hypertension and dyslipidaemia is thought to be a major underlying factor in the increased mortality from coronary heart disease in South Asians. McKeigue and colleagues[4] in a survey of nearly 4000 people in London found that, in comparison to Europeans, South Asians had a higher prevalence of diabetes (19% vs 4%), higher blood pressures, higher fasting and post-glucose insulin concentrations, higher plasma triglycerides and lower HDL cholesterol concentrations. Mean waist–hip girth ratios were also higher in South Asians. This central obesity and insulin resistance are of especial note. However, there are many other factors including smoking, poverty and a higher prevalence of a broad range of other non-biochemical risk factors in South Asian patients compared to the general population.

Although the prevalence of diabetes in patients of Indian, Pakistani and Bangladeshi origin is similar there are important differences in the risk of coronary heart disease between these groups. Therefore strategies to control coronary heart disease in South Asians should emphasize all important established factors specific to different ethnic backgrounds. Furthermore, migrants from the Indian sub-continent to the UK have less favourable coronary risk profiles compared to their siblings who do not migrate. However, the UK Prospective Diabetes Study has shown that treatment of blood pressure and glycaemic control can lead to reduction in cardiovascular complications.

Other complications of diabetes

The few studies on complication rates for diabetes in patients of ethnic minority communities have been limited to those in secondary care. Glycated haemoglobin levels are higher in South Asian people with diabetes attending hospital clinics than they are in indigenous white populations.[5] Although the prevalence of coronary heart disease is higher in South Asian populations, the prevalence of peripheral vascular disease and subsequent ulceration and amputation are rare in South Asian patients with diabetes. South Asians are also less likely to have retinopathy. The reasons for this are unclear.

The prevalence of proteinuria and microalbuminuria is higher among South Asian people with diabetes than in white people.[5] South Asians and African-Caribbean people also have higher prevalence of end-stage renal disease. They have 3–4-fold higher acceptance rates on renal dialysis replacement therapy than white people. Key reasons include difficulties in tissue matching and shortage of donor organs. There appears to be a reduced willingness for organ donation in South Asian groups, which may be due to religious or cultural resistance. However, with education and the support of community leaders this is changing. A recent TV campaign to find bone marrow donors for a young child was very successful, suggesting that resistance to organ donation can be overcome. Primary care professionals will also have a key role in raising awareness of lack of donor organs.

Prevention of diabetes

Type 2 diabetes is a lifestyle-related disease and can be prevented or delayed by lifestyle interventions. This is particularly relevant to South Asians (the prevalence of diabetes is low in rural communities in the Indian sub-continent). The key interventions for prevention of diabetes are increasing physical activity and reducing obesity. Interventions regarding this are discussed in Chapter 11. Key issues include raising awareness among South Asian communities and increased access to physical activity and dietary advice.

Care of diabetes

Successful management requires that the people delivering care understand the lifestyles, attitudes and beliefs of the person with diabetes. People from ethnic minority communities may not get the services that they need because of differences in language, literacy and culture.[6] Furthermore, knowledge about diabetes and risk factors for coronary heart disease are poorer in people from ethnic minority communities.[6] The care of individuals will need to be tailored to their individual needs (see Box 12.1).

Box 12.1 **Needs of people with diabetes from ethnic minority communities**

- Availability and use of appropriate language and translation services
- Exploration of patient's beliefs and behaviours or barriers to health promotion or care
- Culturally specific health educational strategies
- Appropriately tailored health promotion programmes including dietary intervention and exercise programmes
- Raise awareness of the increased risk of complications, in particular cardiovascular complications such as CHD
- Advice on importance of tight glycaemic and blood pressure control

Most translation occurs through family members. Bilingual interpreters, link workers and advocates have tended to be underused, although it is important to work with them where appropriate in order to improve effective communication and quality of care, as considered in Chapters 3, 7 and 8.

In one study quite varied beliefs and behaviours were identified among British Bangladeshis with diabetes. Many structural and material barriers to improving health were identified, including poor housing, unsafe streets, religious restrictions and financial hardship. Bangladeshi patients also indicated a higher regard for verbal explanations from informal sources including friends, relatives and other patients with diabetes. Exploring individuals' beliefs, attitudes and behaviours will be important in promoting good diabetes care and wider health promotion programmes.[7]

Some South Asians may use various herbal and natural remedies for the treatment of diabetes. These include karela, fenugreek, garlic and bitter gourds which are frequently taken for treatment of diabetes.[5] These patients need to be given appropriate advice and education to avoid relying solely on those therapies and to continue their prescribed medications. Often patients have been encouraged to adhere to dietary regimes which are impossible to fit in with their health beliefs and religious beliefs. Culturally appropriate health education and support is required, including written materials and video packages as literacy rates have been found to be low in some cultures.

Fasting during religious festivals

For certain groups of people from South Asia, religious practices such as fasting may sometimes conflict with recommended medical management of diabetes. Many of the world's religions recommend periods of fasting or abstinence from certain foods. Devout Muslims follow the instructions of Allah to fast from sunrise to sunset for a lunar calendar month during Ramadan.[8] The abstention includes all food and drink including water. In the UK, a fast can last 10 hours when Ramadan falls during the winter months, but up to 19 hours in the summer.

People with chronic illness, including diabetes, may be exempted from fasting. Nevertheless, many Muslim people with diabetes will fast to meet their religious obligations. Fasting during Ramadan with oral medication or insulin may potentially lead to hypoglycaemia or ketoacidosis. Many patients will be able to fast safely with appropriate education and counselling, without any clinical complications. Patients need to be educated about warning symptoms of dehydration, hypoglycaemia and hyperglycaemia. They also need to be educated about breaking fasts and seeking immediate medical help during any complications.

Patients on oral hypoglycaemic drugs should reverse their doses so the morning dose is taken before the sunset meal and the evening dose with the morning (pre-sunrise) meal.[8] Long-acting sulphonylureas should be avoided in patients who fast. Patients on insulin can use short-acting insulin before the sunset and sunrise meals with intermediate insulin in the evening.[8]

Hinduism also has many religious festivals during which devotees will fast from periods of 1 day up to 1 month. Similar instructions on adjusting medications before meals should be given.

Improving diabetes services

The Audit Commission has suggested the requirements for an appropriate diabetes service for people from ethnic minority communities (Box 12.2).[6]

Those responsible for caring for people with diabetes within primary care organizations need to be aware of and identify the ethnic composition and language needs of patients within their practices (see Chapter 4). This will identify the interpreting and translation services that will be required alongside the need for link workers and advocates (see Chapters 7 and 8). Previously there have also been calls for the development of diabetes registers for British Asian and African-Caribbean patients with diabetes in the UK,[5] however, coordination and maintenance of such a register would be a difficult task. The development of good practice on patient profiling may enable ethnic specific data from general datasets.

Examples of good models of care are now emerging. A primary care trust (PCT) in Birmingham serves a highly deprived population with 64% of people

---

Box 12.2 **A good diabetes service for people from ethnic minority communities**

The service should:

- have information on the ethnic make-up of its population and target resources accordingly
- be aware of languages spoken, literacy rates, dietary practices, alternative remedies and religious practices
- have sought out views on the service provided
- have appointed staff to reflect the ethnic population, where possible, and train all staff on cultural and religious aspects of diabetes care
- have an accessible and well-used interpreting service
- provide translations of basic literature, such as the Diabetes UK leaflet *What to Expect* and appropriate audiotapes
- have a policy for detecting diabetes in high-risk groups
- give advice on matters such as diet which is sensitive to cultural differences
- monitor outcomes by ethnic groups
- be making attempts to increase awareness of diabetes among high-risk groups.

(*Source*: Audit Commission[6])

of South Asian or African-Caribbean origin[9] and a prevalence of diabetes of around 6%. A previous needs analysis had shown care of people with diabetes to be poor. In response to this the PCT developed a well-organized community diabetes service underpinned by appropriate education, resources and clinical support.

Primary care organizations need to consider the educational needs of primary health care teams in relation to diabetes care. One key component in the Birmingham PCT service is the mandatory attendance for one general practitioner and one practice nurse from each practice at a university-accredited course leading to the Certificate in Primary Care Diabetes. The aim of the course is to extend knowledge, increase skills and develop attitudes towards primary diabetes care for course participants. The course comprises 30 hours of contact time with assessed course work, including an audit, a project, putting learning into practice and a patient case study. There is also a written examination at the end of the course for all candidates. An evaluation of the course showed that there were improvements in the knowledge of health care professionals 1 year after the course. Furthermore, there were reported improvements in organization of diabetes care.

There is a dearth of ethnic-specific diabetes training for health care professionals, and such programmes need to be developed in the UK. Primary care organizations with ethnic populations will have to consider innovative methods for informing patients with diabetes, including a centralized telephone helpline in different languages. These organizations also need to consider developing resource packs to include information on medication, fasting, smoking cessation and prevention of complications.

Innovative methods may need to be used to improve education about diabetes among people from ethnic minority backgrounds. One previous study has shown that a structured pictorial teaching programme for Pakistani Muslim patients with type 2 diabetes resulted in increased knowledge and self-caring behaviour. However, attitudinal views were more resistant to change with patients finding it difficult to choose suitable foods at social occasions. Nevertheless, it appeared the health education programme empowered Asian diabetics to take control of their diets, learn to monitor and interpret glucose results and understand the implications of poor glycaemic control for diabetic complications.[10]

The concepts of 'expert patients' or 'peer educators' are exciting. Project Dil in Leicester has successfully used peer educators in primary prevention of CHD and cardiac rehabilitation (see Chapter 11). These programmes can and should be extended to people with diabetes from minority ethnic communities.

Conclusion

There is currently great opportunity to improve the quality of primary care for people from diverse communities (discussed in Chapter 3). Primary care organizations whose populations include ethnic minority communities need to learn from others that have successfully reconfigured their services to provide appropriate health care of diabetes among minority groups. Examples of new models of care for people from ethnic minority communities are now available for PCTs. At the same time practitioners should remember that, as with any patient of whatever background, effective management means identifying and responding to an individual patient's differing needs and contexts.

Key points

♦ The prevalence of diabetes and impaired glucose tolerance is much higher in certain ethnic groups, including South Asians and African-Caribbeans

♦ Mortality from heart disease is much higher in South Asian patients with diabetes compared to their white British counterparts

♦ The prevalence of other complications of diabetes, including proteinuria, end-stage renal disease, and poor glycaemic control are also higher in South Asian people with diabetes

♦ New innovative models of care will be required to improve care of people with diabetes from ethnic communities

References

1. Simmons D, Williams DRR, Powell MJ. The Coventry Diabetes Study: prevalence of diabetes and impaired glucose tolerance in Europids and Asians. *Quarterly Journal of Medicine* 1991; 81: 1021–1030.
2. Odugbesan O, Rowe B, Fletcher J, Walford S, Barnett AH. Diabetes in the UK West Indian community: the Wolverhampton survey. *Diabetic Medicine* 1989; 6: 48–52.
3. Chaturvedi N, Fuller JH. Ethnic differences in mortality from cardiovascular disease in the UK: Do they persist in people with diabetes? *Journal of Epidemiology and Community Health* 1996; 50: 137–139.
4. McKeigue PM, Shah B, Marmot MG. Relation of central obesity and insulin resistance with high diabetes prevalence and cardiovascular risk in South Asians. *Lancet* 1991; 337: 382–386.
5. Hopkins A, Bahl V. *Access to health care for people from black and ethnic minorities.* London: Royal College of Physicians of London, 1993.
6. Audit Commission. *Testing times: a review of diabetes services in England and Wales.* London: Audit Commission, 2000.
7. Greenhalgh T, Helman C, Chowdhury AM. Health beliefs and folk models of diabetes in British Bangladeshis: a qualitative study. *BMJ* 1998; 316: 978–983.
8. Shaikh S, James D, Morrissey J, Patel V. Diabetes care and Ramadan: to fast or not to fast? *British Journal of Diabetes and Vascular Disease* 2001; 1: 65–67.

9. Hearnshaw H, Hopkins J, Wild A, MacKinnon M, Gadsby R, Dale J. Mandatory, multidisciplinary education in diabetes care. Can it meet the needs of primary care organisations? *Practical Diabetes International* 2001; 18: 274–280.
10. Hawthorne K, Tomlinson S. One-to-one teaching with pictures – flashcard health education for British Asians with diabetes. *British Journal of General Practice* 1997; 47: 301–304.

Further information

Ahmad WIU (ed.) *Ethnicity, disability and chronic illness.* Buckingham: Open University Press, 2000.

Bhopal R, Unwin N, White M, Yallop J, Walker L, Alberti KG *et al.* Heterogeneity of coronary heart disease risk factors in Indian, Pakistani, Bangladeshi, and European origin populations: cross sectional study. *BMJ* 1999; 319: 215–220.

Burden AC, Samanta A, Rahman F. Customs, mores and diabetes: Lessons from the Indian diabetic. *Practical Diabetes* 1991; 8: 224–226.

Diabetes UK (*http://www.diabetesuk.org.uk*) provides helpful information for health professionals and patients.

Raleigh VS. Diabetes and hypertension in Britain's ethnic minorities: implications for the future of renal services. *BMJ* 1997; 314: 209–213.

13 Hypertension and stroke

Louise Hammersley

Hypertension is common among almost all populations. It is a major risk factor for stroke, which is an extremely important cause of disability and death in all ethnic minority populations. However, these conditions warrant particular attention in people of black or African-Caribbean origin. This chapter outlines aspects of screening and health promotion, and emphasizes important practical issues in the clinical management of hypertension in this group.

Patterns of disease

Hypertension occurs very frequently in people of African-Caribbean origin with a prevalence as high as 50% over the age of 40 years. This is associated with a high incidence of cerebrovascular and renal complications[1,2] (see Box 13.1).

There is no scientific consensus about why the African-Caribbean population is at such high risk of hypertension and stroke. The answer is likely to be multifactorial, but the following are some areas of importance to consider.

Box 13.1   **Risks of hypertension and stroke in African-Caribbean communities**

- The risk of stroke and death from stroke among African-Caribbean people is approximately double that of the general population.
- End-stage renal failure is 20 times more common in black hypertensives as compared to other ethnic groups.
- Black people are more likely to develop left ventricular hypertrophy (LVH). Black patients with mild hypertension have a two-fold higher rate of LVH than non-blacks with similar blood pressure levels.
- Overall among men, the death rate from hypertensive disease is four times greater than the national average. Among women, mortality is seven times greater.

Severity of disease

There is some evidence that black people have a higher incidence of severe hypertension than other groups. The West Midlands Malignant Hypertension Register has shown a higher rate of malignant hypertension, higher blood pressures and more severe renal impairment at presentation. There was also a lower median survival and an increased rate of progression to dialysis.[3]

Pathophyisology

The physiological control of blood pressure is complex, and beyond the scope of this chapter. However, there are some important physiological differences relevant to the treatment of hypertension in the black population. The most important is that black patients with high blood pressure tend to have lower levels of plasma rennin activity and are said to have more salt-sensitive blood pressure responses. Black patients also have greater plasma volumes than the white population. In addition, there is an association between reduced sodium-potassium ATPase activity and hypertension in black patients.[1]

Environmental and social factors

Blood pressure profiles have been found to vary with degree of urbanization, a higher prevalence of hypertension often being observed in urban populations.[4] Living in an urban environment, as the vast majority of the UK African-Caribbean population do, adds a number of unquantifiable stresses such as difficulties in access to health care, exposure to discrimination, or stress related to social disadvantage and poverty.

There is currently interest in examining the role of racism in the aetiology of hypertension. In one US-based study, differences in rates of hypertension between black and white respondents were substantially reduced by taking into account reported experiences of and responses to racial harassment.[5] The reasons for this are not clear, and the influence of social class clouds the issue.

Access to health care and concordance with treatment

A survey conducted by the Health Education Authority in 1994 showed that among the younger age groups of African-Caribbean men only 3% visited their GP compared to 7% of the UK population as a whole. This has obvious consequences for the opportunistic detection and subsequent treatment of hypertension.

Practitioners should also explore patients' beliefs and understandings about hypertension. One qualitative study with patients in the African-Caribbean population has shown that concordance with pharmacological treatment may be low, due to a belief in the efficacy of herbal treatment. There was also a perception that high blood pressure is normal.[6] This seems understandable, given the high prevalence and common experience of hypertension in this community.

Management of hypertension in African-Caribbean populations

The various aspects to treatment that are particular to black patients with hypertension are outlined below.

Non-pharmacological management

Changes in lifestyle can cause significant drops in blood pressure in black patients.

Salt restriction

There is evidence that salt restriction (to <100 mmol daily) is as effective as low-dose thiazide diuretics in mild to moderate hypertension. In those without evidence of target organ damage (i.e. proteinuria, renal impairment, left ventricular hypertrophy, heart failure, stroke, transient ischaemic attack, hypertensive eye disease or peripheral vascular disease), a low-salt diet may occasionally be enough to control blood pressure.[7] In addition a low-potassium diet has been found to be common in black patients with hypertension, and increased dietary intake (to 100–120 mmol daily) has been shown to have an added anti-hypertensive effect, particularly in people in lower socio-economic groups.

Weight control

Studies have shown that in black people with hypertension there is a high prevalence of obesity, with a mean weight approximately 20–25% above healthy levels. Weight loss may not have as much effect on blood pressure as in white patients, but it should nonetheless be encouraged.[1]

Other lifestyle change

As for all hypertensives, advice about smoking, exercise and alcohol consumption should be given. There is no data comparing the effects of these measures in different ethnic groups, but such advice is accepted good practice. As already noted, it is important to ask about patient's use of herbal remedies, which some patients may use in preference to prescribed medication.

Pharmacological treatment

There are some important considerations for drug treatment of hypertension among black patients.

Diuretics

Low-dose thiazide diuretics should be first line treatment in most black patients. They cause a greater drop in blood pressure in black patients than in white patients. This is likely to be due to the increased salt sensitivity, low renin activity, reduced Na^+/K^+-ATPase activity and relative expansion of the blood volume. At low doses metabolic disturbances are very rare, but diuretics can have detrimental effects on lipid profiles and glycaemic control and should be used carefully in patients with such problems.

♦ Diuretics should be used as first line treatment.

Beta-blockers

Beta-blockers are generally not as effective in black as in white hypertensives. This is because of their low renin status, combined with a generally lower cardiac output and high peripheral resistance. However, if they are used in combination with a drug that activates the renin-angiotensin system, that is diuretics, calcium antagonists, or alpha-blockers, patients may respond. Young patients may be more responsive than older patients, as renin levels drop with age.

It should also be noted that erectile dysfunction is a very common side effect with beta-blockers. The effect is dose related and as black patients often end up on large doses, due to their reduced responsiveness, it is of particular relevance to black male patients to take a sexual history.

♦ Unless there is a clear indication (e.g. after myocardial infarction) then beta-blockers should not be used alone as first-line therapy.

Angiotensin-converting enzyme inhibitors

Because of low renin levels and salt sensitivity, black people are also less sensitive to the effects of angiotensin-converting enzyme (ACE) inhibitors. This can again be eliminated by the concomitant use of a diuretic, calcium channel blocker, or alpha-blocker. Studies have shown that a black patient would require two to four times the dose of an ACE inhibitor used alone to gain similar results.[8]

The serious and potentially life-threatening condition of ACE-inhibitor-induced angioedema is more common in black patients, due to hypersensitivity to bradykinin. One study showed an adjusted relative risk of 4.5 in African-Americans.[9] The symptoms usually begin in the first few weeks of therapy, and patients should be warned to report any urticarial symptoms and stop treatment if their lips, face or tongue begins to swell. However, the condition is very rare and the potential benefits of treatment in some cases should be balanced against this.

Due to the same mechanism, cough, a recognized side effect of ACE inhibitors, is more common in black patients. This contributes further to the poor toleration of this class of drug in this patient group. However, ACE inhibitors should continue to be used for renal protection in diabetic patients, particularly those with proteinuria.

◆ Unless there is a clear indication (e.g. diabetic renal disease) ACE inhibitors should not be used as first-line monotherapy.

Calcium channel blockers

Calcium channel blockers are highly effective treatment in black hypertensives. The efficacy of this class of drug is enhanced by the low-renin state. They also have a protective effect on the kidneys because of their vasodilating properties.

◆ Calcium channel blockers should be used alone or with diuretics.

Alpha blockers

By reducing peripheral resistance alpha-blockers can reduce blood pressure in black hypertensives. However, their effects can be inconsistent, as they do not treat the expanded blood volume that black patients have and the addition of a diuretic is often required. They have the advantage of being metabolically neutral and have no effect on lipids or glucose levels.

◆ Alpha-blockers should be considered, but only used in combination with a diuretic.

Angiotensin receptor antagonists

Most of the research done so far on this group of drugs has been on white populations. Their place in the treatment of black patients is as yet unclear.

Drug combinations

Current guidelines from the British Hypertension Society (BHS) advocate the use of lower dose drug combinations than maximal dose of a single agent, as submaximal doses of two drugs result in larger blood pressure responses and fewer side effects than maximal doses of a single drug.

◆ In resistant hypertension in black patients the BHS suggest that a combination of diuretic, calcium antagonist, ACE inhibitor and/or alpha-blocker is particularly effective.

Aspirin

Aspirin has been shown to reduce cardiovascular events with respect to both secondary prevention (patients who already have a confirmed diagnosis of myocardial infarction, angina, coronary artery bypass graft or angioplasty, non-haemorrhagic cerebrovascular disease, peripheral vascular disease or atherosclerotic renovascular disease) and primary prevention under the following circumstances:

◆ blood pressure controlled to <150/90 mmHg **and** aged >50 years **and** target organ damage

or

◆ a 10-year CHD risk of >15% (see below)

or

◆ type 2 diabetes

Statins

The use of statins is currently being targeted at patients in the following circumstances:

◆ for secondary prevention

◆ in patients with a 10-year cardiovascular risk of >30% (see below)

◆ familial hypercholesterolaemia

Box 13.2   **Summary of pharmacological management**

◆ Low-dose thiazides and calcium channel blockers should be first line treatment in black hypertensives
◆ Beta-blockers and ACE inhibitors should not be used as monotherapy, but in combination with another drug to activate the renin–angiotensin system have effects comparable to those in white patients
◆ ACE inhibitors should be considered for patients with co-existing diabetes
◆ Alpha-blockers are most effective if used in combination with a diuretic
◆ Angiotensin receptor antagonists have no been fully assessed in this patient group
◆ Consider aspirin and lipid lowering in those patients at high risk

---

Prevention, health promotion and education

There are no specific guidelines for the care of black populations in the UK. However, issues to consider are the following.

Information

One of the most important activities for health care professionals is to make communities aware of any particular risks they may face. Without this knowledge, individuals are denied the chance to take precautions against the potential harms. At present there is no health promotion information targeted particularly at black populations. It is therefore up to individual practitioners to ensure that they are providing adequate care to their patients.

Screening

The particular importance of screening for hypertension in African-Caribbean communities is obvious. Vigilance in ensuring that all patients over 18 years of age have a blood pressure check is of vital importance. There is no consensus on the regularity with which black patients should have their blood pressure checked, but the general guidance in the British Hypertension Guidelines suggest that checking blood pressure every 5 years in all adult patients until the age of 80 years is good practice.

Lifestyle advice

As previously stated, advice regarding salt restriction and weight loss should be stressed for this group of patients. This may involve referral to a dietitian and advice about local sports facilities.

All patients who smoke should be offered counselling, support and nicotine replacement.

Evidence-based practice

The British Hypertension Society laid down the currently accepted gold standard for the treatment of hypertension in 1999.[7] The recommendations made are based on current research evidence. The issues involved in the care of ethnic groups are considered briefly, but the general information about the management of hypertension apply to all patients. A brief summary is given below.

The aims of treatment

The objective of all interventions is to reduce the incidence of the complications of hypertension. Optimum suggested target blood pressures for antihypertensive treatment are (both the systolic and diastolic pressures should be attained):

	Clinic blood pressure (mmHg)	
	No diabetes	Diabetes
Optimal blood pressure	<140/85	<140/80
Audit standard	<150/90	<140/85

Full screening for complications at diagnosis

All hypertensive patients should have a full history and physical examination at diagnosis, along with a limited number of investigations to exclude target organ damage (renal impairment, LVH, cardiovascular or cerebrovascular disease).

Routine investigations should be limited to:

- urinalysis for blood and protein
- serum creatinine and electrolytes
- blood glucose
- serum total: HDL cholesterol
- ECG.

The information gained should be used to calculate each patient's 10-year cardiac risk, using the computer programme 'Cardiac Risk Assessor' or the CHD risk chart issued by the Joint British Societies.

Early referral

Because of the high levels of complications in black patients at diagnosis, doctors should have a low threshold for referral. In particular, 24-hour blood pressure monitoring for those resistant to treatment, and echocardiography for evaluation of LVH, can be useful. Any indication of renal complications should also trigger referral for a specialist opinion.

Stroke

Once a cerebrovascular event has occurred, the management is the same as for any patient. Initially strokes are best managed in a stroke unit, where specialist care and rehabilitation can be provided.

Once back under community care then a multidisciplinary approach should be adopted, involving for example physiotherapists, occupational therapists, social workers and psychologists, as appropriate.

Medical care should focus on coordination of care and secondary prevention. Careful control of blood pressure, anticoagulation (with aspirin or warfarin as appropriate), lipid lowering and glycaemic control are paramount.

Key points

Among people from African-Caribbean communities:

- There is a high risk of hypertension and its complications
- Raising community awareness of hypertension and screening for hypertension are of heightened importance

- Lowering of dietary salt intake appears particularly valuable
- Some drug treatments appear less effective, and some much more so, in managing hypertension
- In general, avoid beta-blockers and ACE inhibitors, and choose thiazides and calcium channel blockers in preference
- Early referral for specialist assessment should be considered, given that a high level of complications at diagnosis is common

References

1. Gibbs CR, Beevers DG, Lip GYH. The management of hypertensive disease in black patients. *Quarterly Journal of Medicine* 1999; 92: 187–192.
2. Health Development Agency. *Hypertension and the Afro-Caribbean community. Guidance for health professionals.* 2002 (see 'Further information').
3. Lip GYH, Beevers M, Beevers DG. Survival and prognosis of 315 patients with malignant-phase hypertension. *Journal of Hypertension* 1995; 13: 915–924.
4. Brownley KA, Hurwitz BE, Schneiderman N. Ethnic variations in the pharmacological and nonpharmcological treatment of hypertension: biopsychological perspective. *Human Biology* 1999; 71(4): 607–639.
5. Krieger N, Sidney S. Racial discrimination and blood pressure: The CARDIA Study of young black and white adults. *American Journal of Public Health* 1996; 86: 1370–1378.
6. Morgan M. The meaning of high blood pressure among Afro-Caribbean and white patients. In: Kelleher D, Hillier S (eds). *Researching cultural differences in health.* London: Routledge, 1996.
7. Ramsey LE, Williams B, Johnston GD, MacGregor GA, Poston L, Potter JF *et al.* Guidelines for management of hypertension: report of the third working party of the British Hypertension Society. *Journal of Human Hypertension* 1999; 13, 569–592. Available online from the British Hypertension Society website (*http://www.hyp.ac.uk/bhs*), which gives the full guideline and risk calculators.
8. Weir MR, Gray JM, Paster R, Saunders E. Differing mechanisms of action of angiotensin-converting enzyme inhibition in black and white hypertensive patients. The Trandolapril Multicentre Study Group. *Hypertension* 1995; 26:124–130.
9. Brown NJ, Ray WA, Snowden M, Griffin MR. Black Americans have an increased rate of angiotensin converting enzyme inhibitor-associated angioedema. *Clinical Pharmacology and Therapeutics* 1996; 60: 8–13.

Further information

Gibbs CR, Beevers DG, Lip GYH. The management of hypertensive disease in black patients. *Quarterly Journal of Medicine* 1999; 92: 187–192. This review article gives more detail on the pathopysiology of hypertension in black people and is a good clear summary of current knowledge.

There is very little information available that is specific to any ethnic group. The Health Development Agency has produced a leaflet on hypertension targeted at the African-Caribbean population in addition to guidance for health professionals, available online at *http://www.hda-online.org.uk*

The following organizations provide general information and patient information leaflets:

British Heart Foundation (*http://www.bhf.org.uk*): Head office: British Heart Foundation, 14 Fitrzhardinge, London, W1H 6DH. Tel: 020 7935 0185 Fax: 020 7486 5820. e-mail: internet@bhf.org.uk

British Hypertension Society Information Service: Blood Pressure Unit, Department of Physiological Medicine, St George's Hospital Medical School, Cramer Terrace, London, SW17 0RE. Tel: 020 8725 3412, Fax: 020 8725 2959, e-mail: bhsis@sghms.ac.uk

Stroke Association (*http://www.stroke.org.uk*). The website gives a full list of all the regional offices.

14 Mental health

Sangeeta Patel

In mental health, more than physical health, the difference between normal and abnormal is determined by context. Whereas physical disorders are assessed by symptoms and signs that denote dysfunction of the body; mental disorders are defined by symptoms and behaviours within a social and cultural context. Psychiatric assessments assume a modern Anglo-European context. (I have used the word 'Anglo-European' throughout this chapter to include British and Northern European. Much also applies to North America.) From that viewpoint, the mental health of people from other ethnic groups is often misunderstood, thus compounding their distress.

In this chapter, I will work from a comment made by a GP to illustrate some of the assumptions on which diagnoses of mental ill health are based, and how they do not necessarily fit people from other ethnic groups.

Interpretations of 'depression'

Towards the end of a study day for GPs in South London about their ethnic minority patients, one GP said,

> The classic [example] that I find most difficult, you were talking about a little earlier, is the lack of, within certain cultures, of the word for depression. So that you find a short fat Asian lady will come in, with her daughter who translates for her and she will have pains through every system in the body and be tired all the time and unable to do anything and in a extreme state, retire herself to bed, with no physical abnormality. As you would say, you would've come out of medical school and you would've examined this lady from top to toe and you would find nothing systemically wrong with her. But you know there is something wrong, and you know how to treat it, but she can't accept your diagnosis or your treatment.
> [Taken from transcripts of GPs discussing their perceived needs on ethnic minority issues; Patel, S. Unpublished work, 2000]

This comment struck a chord with the other GPs present. That study day was attended by 12 GPs, mostly South Asian. They told anecdotes of 'Asian' patients who did not understand 'depression', and consequently refused to take antidepressants or attend counsellors. In a practice in West London, GPs were reported to have recognized as depressed only 17% of the 30% of Indian women found to be depressed by a questionnaire.[1] Asian patients rarely presented symptoms of depression to their GPs. An editorial in the *British Medical Journal* suggested,

> An additional reason for low presentation rates for mental illness is that ideas of psychological causation of illness are poorly understood within Asian cultures.[2]

In 1980, Leff, a prominent psychiatrist developed an evolutionary scale for societies, based on the language they used to express dysphoria.[3] At the bottom of this scale he put those societies with languages that did not differentiate between physical and psychological experiences. At the top, he put those with a range of psychological vocabulary. By emphasizing the number of words that people used to express emotion, rather than other ways in which emotion was expressed, Leff linked psychological vocabulary to 'developed' people. He also linked somatization to 'underdeveloped' people. More recently, this view was echoed by a professor of transcultural psychiatry, to explain the high rates of somatization among South Asians.

> The received wisdom is that people in rural non-Western cultures are not psychologically minded and do not have abstract language or concepts of emotional distress, and therefore communicate their emotions somatically.[4]

Assumptions about 'depression'

The above interpretations are underpinned by several assumptions. 'Depression' is like a disease, and is the 'real' diagnosis. 'Depression', in the form described by psychiatry, is common to all people, regardless of their culture. The failure to understand depression by some cultures results in somatic expression. In the biomedical literature, these assumptions are presented as if they are neutral. Indeed, to those who share the cultural history of psychiatry, these interpretations are common sense. However, to people from other ethnic groups who do not share this cultural history, such biomedical interpretations may not make any sense.

Psychiatric disorders across history and culture

This section focuses on 'depression' to exemplify how particular trains of thought in European cultural history since the 17th century have contributed to psychiatric perspectives.

Depression as an individual mental disorder

In 1637, Descartes distinguished the soul, as the site of thought and feeling, from the body, which was material, mechanical and without a will of its own.

Dissections of the dead body, as the model for the live body, confirmed this viewpoint. The failure to find where the soul resided contributed to the notion of both body and mind as machines. By the 20th century, thought and feeling had been reattributed to the mind.[5] Whereas in 1621, Burton wrote of 'melancholia' as the battle between God and the Devil for man's soul, for Freud in the 20th century, 'melancholia' was located in the individual psyche.

In other cultures, distress has not been so localized to the minds of individuals. In ayurveda (a medical system originating in India around 2000 years ago and widely practised today), for example, mind is of the same substance as the body, although its more subtle form. Health and disease of both mind and body are caused by three humours within and around the body. Hence, 'state of mind' is intimately bound with the rest of the body and its environment, rather than neurochemical processes in the brain, for example.

Depression as a disease

In Europe until the 17th century, imbalances between four humours were thought to cause ill health. Imbalances were caused by individual tendencies as well as environmental circumstances. In 1675, Sydenham proposed a description of diseases, categorized like species, with characteristic symptoms and natural history. Dissection of corpses helped to locate diseases in a more concrete way, with typical features, regardless of the body they occupied. Following Sydenham's lead, academic clinicians began to concentrate their efforts on the discovery of diseases. By the early 19th century, French and English clinicians had worked to develop a catalogue of diseases, each recognizable by characteristic clinical features, often a visible lesion, and ideally a single definite cause. Asylums provided fertile ground for development of psychiatric theories along the same lines. Kraepelin in Germany, Pinnel and Charcot in France, and later Maudsley in England, meticulously described their observations of the mad and melancholic, refining natural histories of diseases from case histories.[6]

From the 1950s, biological psychiatry was propelled into the foreground by the discovery and promotion of psychotropic drugs. Clinical trials to confirm the efficacy of new drugs required standard simple definitions of psychiatric disorders, such as those provided by the American Psychiatric Association's *Diagnostic and Statistical Manual for Mental Disorders*, now in its fourth edition. By 1980, 10 million prescriptions of antidepressants were issued in the USA yearly, and pharmaceutical companies came only after the arms industry in international trade. Depression was not confined to hospitals and entered the public domain, with prevalence rates reported as high as 1 in 10 in England in 2001.

Psychiatric disorders, as diseases, became the focus of the biomedical gaze. To doctors, the symptoms were of more interest than individual patient's circumstances that led to their distress. The key symptoms of psychiatric disorders were based on European experiences. For example, the subjective feeling of sinking down – 'depression' and 'low mood' came into common currency during the economic downturn in England and America in the 1930s;[7] 'fatigue' alongside the rise of the protestant work ethic and 'guilt', associated with sickness as a prominent feature of Christendom from the middle ages. Worldwide, 'soul loss' better describes the experience than 'depression'. 'Shame' is more frequent than 'guilt' in many South Asian people.

Depression 'somatized'

Disorders in which patients experience both physical and mental symptoms create a particular tension in biomedicine. With many physical diseases, the doctor's interpretation can be confirmed or refuted by further investigations. Without a physical cause, doctors attribute symptoms to mental disorders, such as 'depression'. When patients don't believe the cause is mental, they are assumed to be 'somatizing'. From another perspective, it is the doctor's 'psychologizing', that is their assumption that the disorder is really psychological, which makes them think that the patient is 'somatizing'. Psychological disorders continue to carry a stigma. 'Somatized' disorders are unpopular with health professionals.

People from cultures in which psyche and soma have not been so deeply divided as in Europe may present symptoms of both to their doctor. They can then find themselves and their whole culture's expressions both pathologized and stigmatized, as shown by the comments from doctors above. In contrast, Nichter described how an ayurvedic practitioner in North India recognized cultural idioms of distress and treated them within their own cultural context, without the shame that a psychological diagnosis would bring.[8]

Psychiatry and race

Psychiatry itself developed in the 19th century, at a time of colonial expansion. Anthropologists then described the physical differences between 'races' (see Chapter 1) and, following trends in biomedicine, used those to explain differences in behaviour and mental capacity. Such differences were interpreted according to European norms and understandings. Patterns of psychosis in other cultures, such as *amok* and *latah*, were interpreted as an underdeveloped form of schizophrenia, for example.[9]

After the Second World War, and the discrediting of eugenic and hierarchical interpretations, many of the locally recognized behavioural disorders in other races or cultures were considered to be 'culture-bound syndromes'. With that exception, there remains the assumption in biological psychiatry that all psychiatric disorders are universal across cultures, in form if not content.[9] (The 'form' of a disorder refers to the type of symptom, such as a delusion; the 'content' to descriptive details, such as seeing Jesus.) That said, diagnoses made in other cultural or racial groups remain in keeping with popular stereotypes; of the African as out of control and the Asian as too controlled, for example.

(African-Caribbeans in Britain are more likely than any other ethnic group to be diagnosed with schizophrenia or other psychosis, forcibly detained under the Mental Health Act, given higher doses of medication and less likely to be referred for psychological treatments.)

Alternative approaches

Over recent years, anthropologists, working from their study of other cultures, have criticized psychiatric approaches. Kleinman outlined how the application of categories from one culture to another in which they did not have meaning committed a 'category fallacy', for example. However, as so much of the academic tradition is also built on the European cultural history outlined above, European interpretations also persist in anthropology. For example, in his study of affective disorders among the Chinese in Taiwan, although Kleinman described the Chinese understandings of health, he still considered the emotional state to be biological, and the cognitive interpretation to be cultural.[10] He thus separated thought and emotion, in keeping with Anglo-European paradigms.

In a study to develop a questionnaire for depression among Punjabis in England, Krause found that although Punjabi people did express more somatic symptoms, they also shared many psychological symptoms with the white British people in the study. Underlying these symptoms lay a markedly different conception of health. For the Punjabis, symptoms were only significant to explain the balance in their bodies of hot and cold, and wet and dry properties.[11]

Krause understood the cultural context, but she described the difficulty she had putting to one side the European constructs that she used to understand the world. For example, she found her view of the ideal cold person, the holy man, was still tinged with her own notions of 'cold' as unfriendly and uncaring. At bottom it is often still the European constructs that have influenced interpretations, albeit less in anthropology than psychiatry.

Other studies have aimed to explore emotions from within indigenous frameworks and the social context. Schieffelin, for example, explains how the Kaluli of Papua New Guinea frame anger and grief within a system of social reciprocity.[12] They undergo a process where the anger and grief are expressed publicly, and thus acknowledged by others and resolved with adequate compensation. He argues how this protects against inward blame, guilt or self-hate. His approach highlights the cultural context within which grief is understood, rather than interpretations that assume emotions are framed psychologically.

Towards more culturally sensitive practice

Recognizing the limits of Anglo-European psychiatry

Biomedical training tends to treat psychiatric categories as fixed, neutral and universal. An understanding of the limited applicability of Anglo-European psychiatric diagnoses may help practitioners to hold back from the tendency in biomedicine to impose those views on people of other cultures.

An appreciation of the role of psychiatry in perpetuating racial stereotypes may prevent practitioners from inadvertently acting on stereotypes or institutional prejudice. Although there may be certain symptoms that people from other cultures have in common with Anglo-European cultures, and they may fit psychiatric categories, neither the symptoms nor the ways they are organized necessarily have the same meaning for the patients. If treatment is to have salience for patients, it must be negotiated with their own frameworks in mind.

Moving from disease to person

The drift in biomedicine over the last four centuries has been to focus on and treat the diseases from which patients suffer. Patients, however, interpret and present symptoms in accordance with their own personal history and ethnic background. These patients are not only vulnerable because of illness, but also because they may not know what is expected of them as patients. It may seem odd to patients that the doctors try to see through the 'content' of symptoms, looking for the 'form', the underlying disease. The patient wants to know the meanings of the symptoms, their cause, the implication on their lives, predictions, and a cure, whereas the doctor wants diagnosis, treatment and prognosis.

In mental health across cultures, the tension is heightened because the worlds of the doctor and patient can be so different. This requires a conceptual shift from the doctor, away from their own preconceptions, towards those of the patient, to appreciate what symptoms mean to the patient in their own world. It may also change the power balance in the consultation, as the doctor needs the patients' knowledge and expertise rather than only their own.

Learning about other medical frameworks

This is potentially the most difficult, and yet most rewarding, aspect of cross-cultural mental health. It requires a critical approach towards biomedical literature, much of which is underpinned by Anglo-European perspectives. For other cultures, relevant literature may lie outside of the medical domain – the trend in modern biomedicine to incorporate mental disorders does not apply to all other medical systems. That said, biomedicine has hegemony the world over: in Britain it would be rare to find people, whatever their ethnic group, whose understanding was not influenced by biomedicine.

This means that doctors have to explore the particular perspective of each patient, assessing how much biomedicine and other cultural understandings bring to bear on their illness. This may seem a tall order, particularly if the aim is to grasp the nuances of every culture. Furthermore, the time constraints in primary care can be seen as a barrier to exploring patients' cultural understandings of illness. That said, the community base and the longer-term continuity of primary care offers the opportunity to get to know the social and cultural conditions of a patient's life. In practices where one ethnic group may be more prominent, knowledge about the cultural understandings of health of that group can save conflict in potentially fraught consultations. Familiarity with the medical frameworks of at least one culture outside biomedicine will enable a more open approach to other ethnic groups, not limited to mental health.

Key points

- The health professional's understanding of the mind, body and disease is limited and may not be shared by patients with a different cultural history
- Patients interpret and present symptoms in accordance with their own personal history and ethnic background
- Some patients are not only vulnerable because of illness, but also because they may not know what is expected of them as patients
- It is the health professional's responsibility to familiarize themselves with their patient's understandings and adjust their practice accordingly
- The aim is to address patients concerns in context, rather than solely treat the mental disorder

References

1. Jacob KS, Bhugra D, Lloyd KR, Mann AH. Common mental disorders, explanatory models and consultation behaviour among Indian women living in the UK. *Journal of the Royal Society of Medicine* 1998; 91: 66–71.
2. Ineichen B. The mental health of Asians in Britain. *BMJ* 1990; 300: 1669–1670.
3. Leff J. *Psychiatry around the globe: a transcultural view.* New York: Marcel Dekker, 1981.
4. Mumford DB, Nazir FJ, Baig IY. Stres and psychiatric disorder in the Hindu Kush. *British Journal of Psychiatry* 1996; 168: 299–307.
5. McDougall W. *Body and mind: a history and defense of animism.* London: Methuen & Co, 1911.
6. Porter R. *Madness: a brief history.* Oxford: Oxford University Press, 2002.
7. Jadhav S. The cultural origins of Western depression. *International Journal of Social Psychiatry* 1996; 42: 269–286.
8. Nichter M. Negotiation of the illness experience: Ayurvedic therapy and the psychosocial dimension of illness. *Culture, Medicine and Psychiatry* 1981; 5: 5–24.
9. Littlewood R. Psychiatry's culture. *International Journal of Social Psychiatry* 1996; 42: 245–265.
10. Kleinman A. *Patients and healers in the context of culture.* Berkeley: University of California Press, 1980.

11. Krause IB. Numbers and meaning: a dialogue in cross-cultural psychiatry. *Journal of the Royal Society of Medicine* 1994; 87: 278–282.
12. Schieffelin EL. The cultural analysis of depressive affect: an example from New Guinea. In Kleinman A, Good BJ (eds). *Culture and depression.* Berkeley: University of California Press, 1985, pp. 101–133.

Further information

Fernando S. *Mental health, race and culture.* London: Mind Publications, 1991. Provides an accessible overview of the impact of racism in psychiatry and considers alternative ways in which to approach mental health in other cultures.

Littlewood R, Dein S. *Cultural psychiatry and medical anthropology: an introduction and reader.* London: Athlone Press, 2000. Brings together influential papers in the development of cultural psychiatry.

Nazroo J. *Ethnicity and Mental Health.* London: Policy Studies Institute, 1997. Reports findings from a national community survey and provides useful discussion on the challenges of their interpretation.

Skultans V, Cox J. *Anthropological approaches to psychological medicine: crossing bridges.* London: Jessica Kingsley, 2000. Explores theoretical and clinical aspects.

15 Care of older people

Greta Rait and Steve Iliffe

The care of older people is complex and challenging, involving physical and psychological co-morbidity, disability and socio-economic factors. Ethnicity, of course, contributes to this picture. Ethnicity is not in itself problematic. It is one way to deepen our understanding of heterogeneity in populations and how this is reflected in health, illness and disability.

This chapter highlights aspects of demography, disadvantage and health beliefs, in considering the response of health care providers to older people from ethnic minorities. It uses the example of mental health to illustrate an approach to care.

Demography

Whereas approximately 16% of the UK population as a whole are over 65, older people from black and ethnic minority groups (BMEGs) make up only 4% of the BMEG population. There were an estimated quarter of a million older people from minority backgrounds in 2000, the majority living in urban, particularly inner city areas. This is expected to increase rapidly over the next two decades, reflecting the pattern and timing of migration. Women start to outnumber men with increasing age and greater numbers of older members of ethnic minorities will live into their seventies and beyond.

Individual needs

Older people from BMEGs have different cultural, religious, and social backgrounds. Within each community there are differences between individuals. These will affect views towards ageing, family care, health and social care. On a community and individual level their interaction with the majority white community will differ. Although they have some common experiences, for example migration and discrimination, they also have different histories, cultural views and beliefs.

Cultural diversity and disadvantage combine together in different ways for different groups. As underscored in Chapter 10, practitioners should avoid seeing older people from BMEGs as 'problem groups', but instead consider specific solutions to specific problems[1] and in particular focus on an individual's needs.

Beliefs and expectations

All societies are influenced by social, political and economic factors, but retain former institutions and cultural beliefs. Following migration there may be a shift in cultural behaviour, with incorporation or modification of some ideas and traditions from the host society.

Initially many migrants expected that their stay in the UK would be temporary, and that they would return home when economically successful. Over time expectations changed, particularly as families settled, creating changes in working patterns and relationship dynamics in many families with potential to cause conflict. As a consequence, life after retirement may not be as originally planned or hoped for. Many older people from ethnic minority backgrounds moved to the UK as young adults. Their own experience of ageing is limited as many left their elderly relatives behind. Their attitudes to ageing are influenced by experiences in their countries of birth and the UK.

Experience of disadvantage

Older people from ethnic minority communities face problems in common with all older people such as social, financial, and health problems as well as issues particular to their ethnic background. They may face the 'double jeopardy' of devaluation in status associated with old age combined with the disadvantages of minority group status, or 'triple jeopardy' including socio-economic disadvantage as well.

Experience of disadvantage may differ. For example, in general, older Pakistanis and Bangladeshis experience greater deprivation than older Indians. Socio-economic disadvantage follows discrimination in housing and employment, job insecurity, low-paid employment, lower pensions and lack of awareness of benefits. They are therefore likely to experience poverty, and the health risks associated with poverty.

Older people from BMEGs are less likely to be fluent or literate in English than younger people, underlining the need for interpreters and bilingual advocates for effective care (Chapters 7 and 8). Communication is further affected by impairments such as hearing or visual problems.

Assumptions about social networks

The assumptions held by society regarding community strength, extended families and support, without the involvement of formal professional structures, are often false. Families that live together do not necessarily provide company or care for older members. Research in India has shown that urbanization, increasingly nuclear families, migration and dual family careers are making the care of older people more of a social challenge.

Research in a variety of immigrant groups have identified multiple stress factors, including a sense of discontinuity between the past and the present, isolation and home sickness, emotional difficulties, disruption to family and family roles, threats to ethnic identity and conflicts of values between the traditional and host culture.

Health care

The health of older people from BMEGs has been inadequately studied (Box 15.1). This makes an evidence based approach to care more difficult but general principles can be drawn from other work with older people.

Care of older people

Disability is the gap between the demands of the environment and the individual's capabilities. Membership of a BMEG may influence disability in several ways. For example, it may be associated with low income and poor access to services due to limited educational opportunity or language barriers. Professionals may have misplaced perceptions of support that the surrounding family or community can or should give.

Box 15.1   Research and older people from BMEGs in the UK

Little research because of:
- **Assumptions**
  Migrants return to their 'homeland'
  Migrants assimilate and have no particular needs
  The numbers are too small ('invisibility of the community')
- **Exclusions**
  Ethnicity and language difficulties are perceived to make research and the interpretation of results difficult.
  Problems with available research:
- **Quality**
  Studies have investigated ethnicity and ignored wider socio-economic contexts
  Studies are difficult because of problems with definitions, recruitment and small numbers
- **Dissemination**
  Studies by local bodies e.g. in the voluntary sector, are not widely disseminated.
  Studies may be published in less accessible specialized journals.

Health and social services

Older people from BMEGs are often under-represented in social and main-stream voluntary services, and may be poorly informed about them. Knowledge and information, communication issues, education about 'rights', together with the appropriateness and acceptability of services, affect pathways to those services and satisfaction with them.

Assumptions by professionals about greater availability of alternative sources of help and support for older people from BMEGs may result in their not being referred to statutory and voluntary services. It may be thought that other help is not welcome, or that the family would rather take care of the older person. This not only limits options for older people from BMEGs but may also militate against further investment in appropriate service development.

As highlighted in Chapter 3, with the exception of the Chinese, people from BMEGs tend to consult their GP with comparable or higher frequency than the general population. This may reflect several factors such as differences in morbidity and need, socio-economic disadvantage, compromised communication or poorer outcomes from consultations. As registration with GPs is high, the primary care team—including health visitors, practice and district nurses – is in a powerful position to facilitate appropriate care and access to wider services. In particular, established relationships between patients and teams may allow for exploration of problems and an awareness of family and carer situations.

Developing and providing primary care

Improving the care of older people in the UK is a government policy priority.[2] The care of older people from BMEGs needs to be based on these standards.

The principles of improving access to care, effective communication with patients, learning to respond effectively to diversity, and care of some common clinical conditions have been discussed in previous chapters.

Strategies for improving services for older people are highlighted in Box 15.2. General issues for enhancing care at practice and community levels are then discussed. The mental health of older people is then considered in more detail.

Improving care at practice level

The consultation

The consultation is key to diagnosing illness and recognizing problems (see Box 15.3). Individuals have their own explanatory models of illness. These need to be explored to understand the presentation of symptoms, reasons for concerns and reactions to diagnosis and management.

Box 15.2   **Strategies to improve services for older people**

- **Local surveys**
  Practice level, e.g. patient satisfaction
  Primary Care Trust level, e.g. needs assessments
- **Data monitoring**
  Service contacts, e.g. attendance, referrals
  Service provision, e.g. blood pressure measurement, cardiac risk
  assessment
- **User representation**
  Representatives from many organizations
  Past and potential service users
  Inclusion of smaller minority groups
  Working in partnership
- **Accessible processes to include users**
  Not threatening or hostile
  Provide feedback
- **Staff training**
  Cultural issues, e.g. diet, death rituals
- **Health improvement days**
  Use community and day centres and religious organizations
  Access to welfare rights advice

Box 15.3   **Key considerations at the consultation**

- Establishing a relationship, e.g. establishing cultural identity,
  availability of interpreters
- Exploring health beliefs
- Social and economic circumstances, e.g. lifestyle factors, social support
  networks
- Assessing for chronic disease, e.g. heart disease, diabetes, hypertension
- Assessing for common problems that impair quality of life, e.g. sensory
  impairment, continence
- Assessing mental health
- Addressing disease, impairments and disability

People's experiences of health services may affect their views on the professional-patient relationship. For example, those who have experienced a paternalistic system may find joint decision-making difficult, or not question any decisions made. There may be expectations of treatment, e.g. injections rather than tablets. Certain symptoms, for example psychological symptoms, may not be considered appropriate to take to the consultation.

Other issues include communication and sensory impairments. Nurse consultations with older people provide the opportunity to gather health and social information and provide a health assessment. Special practice clinics with interpreters have been used to encourage older people to attend and focus on their needs.

Apparently straightforward problems have different meanings for different cultures. For example, urinary frequency may suggest infection, diabetes or detrusor instability to the doctor or nurse. However, the professional may be unaware of the issues of privacy, hygiene and religious observance that are more salient to some Hindus, Sikhs and Muslims.

Reviewing practice

Primary care practices can assess their structures and processes to see if there are barriers to accessing services. This should include reviewing availability of appropriate practice information, procedures for making appointments, reception procedures and repeat prescriptions, and bilingual staff members reflecting the local community (see Chapters 3, 5 and 10). Some practices hold open days with interpreters and community workers present to explain procedures, as well as providing preventative care and health education.

The crucial importance of recording patients' ethnicity has been underlined in Chapter 4. This can enable development of more culturally sensitive services, provide information to support requests for additional resources such as interpreting services, and assist in identifying individuals at greater risk from certain chronic diseases such as diabetes.

Variations in care for different groups of patients may not be noticed if only the whole practice or total locality population is considered. Practices recording patients' ethnicity should use clinical audit to establish if patients from different ethnic groups are receiving similar standards of care, for example of their diabetes or heart disease.

Coordination of care

Care of chronic diseases and complex needs requires well coordinated multidisciplinary care, across primary, secondary and residential care and social services. There are two traps for the unwary: making assumptions about how need is being met, and making assumptions about how symptoms and disabilities are experienced.

Assumptions made about the care-giving capacity of existing support systems for individuals from minority ethnic groups may lead to differences in service utilization. For example:

♦ Low uptake of community health and social services by ethnic minority elders may be seen by white GPs as evidence of care by the extended family and by Asian GPs as evidence of language barriers, limited knowledge of services and poor service response.[3]

♦ Assumptions about family care made by gatekeepers may explain the under-representation of older black people on community nurse caseloads in the Midlands[4] and the under-utilization of services for leg ulcers by ethnic minority elders in West London.[5]

Improving care for communities

Development of partnerships and user involvement are key. Many community and voluntary organizations have arisen because mainstream services have failed to provide suitable services for minority elders. These services often provide support and information that cannot be found in the statutory sector. They include day centres, residential homes, or facilities based in religious organizations.

Primary care trusts (PCTs) need to identify these services and organizations, and learn from them by developing partnerships. User involvement is important in this process but methods of doing so need to be accessible and non-threatening. This also needs to include a variety of community groups in order to be representative of a locality.

At a PCT level, ethnicity profiling can assist in the commissioning of services, for example stroke services, interpreting services, health advocates or link workers. Emphasis should be on including older people who may encounter barriers to providing this information, e.g. those with language, visual or hearing impairments.

Older people and mental health

A broad perspective on mental health and cultural diversity is provided in Chapter 14. Here we concentrate on the particular challenges and high prevalence of depression and dementia among older people. Up to 16% of older people experience depressive symptoms, and the overall prevalence of dementia is 4–7%. The National Service Framework for Older People states that ethnic minority communities need accessible and appropriate mental health services, but does not expand on how this will be achieved.

Depression

Prevalence and incidence of mental health problems among BMEGs are difficult to calculate because of inaccurate or inadequate data, people not presenting to services, and difficulties with detection, diagnosis and cross-cultural understanding. Older South Asians and African-Caribbeans may associate stress such as racism, unemployment and financial difficulties with depression.

Language problems are often cited as reasons for not detecting psychological distress. Using family members as interpreters is self-evidently unsuitable (Chapters 7 and 8), but it is difficult to arrange a trained interpreter for all encounters with patients. Moreover, although there are similarities in patterns of depression across cultures, there are also complex differences in presentation, language used and symptoms reported that need careful exploration by practitioners. For example a survey of 209 Punjabi and 180 white English patients attending general practices in London[6] showed that:

♦ Punjabi patients with depressive ideas were less likely to be detected than white English ones.

♦ The prevalence of common mental disorders was not influenced by culture. Punjabi individuals scoring as depressed on the Amritsar Depression Inventory and the General Health Questionnaire often had 'poor concentration and memory' and 'depressive ideas' but – contrary to common stereotypes – were not more likely to have somatic symptoms.

♦ GPs were more likely to assess Punjabis with common mental disorder as having 'physical or somatic symptoms' or 'sub-clinical disorders'.

Misunderstanding concepts and meanings

A simplistic view of how ethnicity might influence an individual's vulnerability to and experience of depression should be avoided. For example, we may take for granted the universality of western concepts such as 'coping mechanisms' or 'social support'. Yet 'social support' for older people in adverse circumstances may mean any of:

♦ help from family and neighbours (particularly among women)

♦ assistance by friends rather than family (particularly among men)

♦ contact with children (particularly in urban populations)

♦ being blessed by ancestors

♦ interaction with a 'compadre'

♦ respecting the precise rules of a complex ritual, particularly with mourning.

Similarly, 'somatization' is easily misunderstood. It is of course common in all communities for psychological complaints to present with physical symptoms. However, in a Chinese community, for example psychological illness may be considered disgraceful and blameworthy, and physical illness an escape route from social stresses. In such a situation, somatization is not a problem but a solution. Attempts to re-attribute a patient's physical symptoms to psychological causes or social stressors may be counter-productive (see further discussion in Chapter 14).

The meaning of experience appears to be central to vulnerability to depression. We do not experience depression in later life simply because life events accumulate, but because events produce losses that are important to individuals in terms of conscious significance (e.g. loss of face), previous difficulties (struggling against a racist culture), or role conflict.

Dementia

General barriers to diagnosis of dementia in the community include not perceiving there is much to offer individuals and carers, lack of definitive diagnosis, difficulties giving the diagnosis, and lack of adequate training to detect and manage mental health. These are accentuated where language and culture may affect presentation and the consultation dynamic. Mild cognitive changes may go unnoticed if older people live with their families, as they are less likely to face financial and domestic challenges.

Identification of cognitive impairment using screening tests relies greatly on language recognition and ability. Different cultures have different patterns of experience, which influence performance. Some screening tests have been validated in ethnic communities (e.g. Mini Mental State Examination in African-Caribbeans).

Evidence-based guidelines are available for the detection[7] and management of dementia in primary care (though there is little specific for BMEGs). Elements of care are largely similar to all communities but include:

- working with interpreters where appropriate
- taking a history of cognitive and behavioural symptoms
- using culturally specific instruments where available
- providing appropriate and accessible information (e.g. audiotapes or videos)
- increasing patient and family awareness and reducing stigma and fear
- seeking specialist assessment and advice
- involving families in formulation of care plans
- accessing the local voluntary sector (e.g. day centres)
- assessing and supporting carers (e.g. by referral to support organizations such as Alzheimer's Society and MIND)
- liaising between primary and secondary old age and other services.

Conclusion

This chapter has highlighted ways of improving quality of care of older people from diverse communities who may experience multiple disadvantage.

Practitioners need to recognize the differing needs of communities and individuals, and review how they can respond appropriately at patient, practice and community levels. Knowledge of the make-up and needs of the local population, and involvement of users and local organizations are essential in shaping appropriate service development.

Key points

◆ The care of older people is complex and challenging, involving physical, and psychological morbidity, disability and socio-economic factors

◆ People from black and ethnic minority groups are diverse and face multiple disadvantages

◆ There is little available evidence on which to base best practice, so practitioners need to work towards achieving nationally set standards

◆ Care should be considered at an individual, practice and community level

◆ Barriers to accessing care need to be identified and addressed

◆ Patient profiling (ethnic monitoring) and user involvement can provide useful information on population make-up and health and social needs

References

1. Atkin K. Ageing in multi-racial Britain: demography, policy and practice. In: Bernard M, Phillips J (eds). *The social policy of old age*. London: Centre for Policy on Ageing, 1998.
2. *National service framework for older people*. London: Department of Health, 2001.
3. Pharoah C. Primary health care for elderly people from black and ethnic minority communities. London: Age Concern Institute of Gerontology/HMSO, 1995.
4. Cameron E, Badger F, Evers H. District nursing, the disabled and the elderly: where are the black patients? *Journal of Advanced Nursing* 1989; 14: 376–382.
5. Franks PJ, Morton N, Campbell A *et al*. Leg ulceration and ethnicity: a study in West London. Public Health 1997; 111: 327–329.
6. Bhui K, Bhugra, Goldberg D, Dunn G, Desai M. Cultural influences on the prevalence of common mental disorder, general practitioners assessments and help-seeking among Punjabi and English people visiting their general practitioner. *Psychological Medicine* 2001; 31(5): 815–825.
7. Eccles M, Clarke J, Livingston M, Freemantle N, Mason J. North of England evidence based guidelines development project; guideline for the primary care management of dementia. *BMJ* 1998; 317: 802–808.

Further information

Hertzman C, Frank J, Evans RG. Heterogeneities in health status and the determinants of population health. In: Evans RG, Barer ML, Marmor TR (eds). *Why are some people healthy and others not?; the determinants of health of populations.* New York: Aldine de Gruyter, 1994.

Iliffe S, Drennan V. *Primary care for older people.* Oxford: Oxford University Press, 2000.

Department of Health (*http://www.doh.gov.uk/race_equality/profiling.htm*): website includes details of primary care and community projects including ethnic monitoring, and an overview of mainstreaming.

Health Development Agency (*http://www.hda-online.org.uk*): examples of publications include *Ethnicity, health and health behaviour: a study of older groups.*

King's Fund (http://www.kingsfund.org.uk).

16 Children and young families

Aziz Sheikh and Abdul Rashid Gatrad

Health at the very beginning of life is the foundation for health throughout life.
(*The NHS Plan*, 2000)

There now exists a considerable body of evidence highlighting the major health inequalities experienced by black and minority ethnic groups (BMEGs) in Britain. Crucial to redressing these inequities is the need to improve the health outcomes of children, for health in the very earliest stages of life represents an important determinant of health status in future life. Research suggests that difficulties in accessing high-quality primary care services are a key factor that disadvantages minority ethnic families. In this chapter, we focus on providing the understanding needed to work with minority ethnic families and on suggesting practical approaches that may usefully improve access to and quality of primary health care services for black and minority ethnic children.

Understanding families from diverse communities

Demographic and socio-economic profile

Almost 1 in 10 children in Britain can now be classified as belonging to a minority ethnic group. Minority ethnic communities are on average younger and have a more unfavourable socio-economic profile than the indigenous white population. The reasons underpinning these important structural and economic differences are readily understood through an awareness of the patterns and dynamics of migration to Britain and familiarity with religious and cultural norms on matters to do with procreation and family life.

Mass migration to Britain is a recent phenomenon, accelerating in the aftermath of the Second World War. A period of rapid industrial and economic growth resulted in labour workforce shortages that attracted young men from the ex-British colonies of Asia and the Caribbean into British inner cities. Migration of dependants (wives, children and parents) followed a decade or two later. More recently migration has continued for political reasons, drawing families from the Balkans, central and western Africa, and South Asia.

Marriage and procreation are strongly encouraged within the indigenous cultures of many migrants. The fertility ratio of such families is on average higher than for white families; acculturation is taking place, however, with evidence suggesting that there is now a trend towards diminishing family size in most ethnic communities.

The strong inter-relationship between deprivation and health outcomes is well known. Ethnic communities are on the whole disadvantaged when compared with white communities. This is to some extent explained by the fact that they represented a labour under-class that initially migrated. Racial and religious discrimination in education, employment and housing opportunities have further compounded this disadvantage (see Chapter 1). Our better appreciation of the association between relative poverty and health outcomes underlines that in order to achieve meaningful progress in tackling health inequalities, urgent action is needed to tackle the wider determinants of health, including, among other things, the need for healthier diets, better housing and improved educational outcomes for children from minority ethnic communities. The government's recently launched Sure Start initiative is one example of a desire to promote social inclusion of marginalized families with young children and address inequality.

Family dynamics and relationships

Acculturation – the phenomenon by which minority cultures gradually adopt the values and ethos of the majority culture – has for many ethnic communities resulted in the erosion of traditional family values. The impact of such accelerated social change, in some cases fracturing cultural narratives sustained over many centuries, can be difficult to fathom for those unfamiliar with religious world-views. Broken marriages, single-parent families and an increasing proportion of children born out of wedlock are just some of the manifestations of an encounter with the secular liberal outlook that now characterizes British society. Such issues pose a particular problem for faith-based communities, many of whom remain reluctant to acknowledge that such problems exist in their midst. The increasing numbers of non-white babies being put up for fostering or adoption, for whom it is proving difficult to find suitable placements, is one consequence of this denial.

Another important consequence of acculturation has been the progressive disintegration of the extended family unit. The lack of readily available expertise of grandparents and other extended family within the household can have important consequences. Those working with such communities may encounter issues that have hitherto typically been dealt with 'in house', including, for example, young mothers attending for advice on breast-feeding, infant feeding and behavioural problems in adolescence.

Improving access to services for children

Flexible and appropriate systems

General considerations for improving access to primary care are discussed in Chapters 3 and 5. Notions of structured pro-active care are a novelty to many people who have recently migrated, particularly those from economically under-developed regions. The observation that surgery and clinic 'Did Not Attend' (DNA) rates are particularly high for many ethnic communities is thus not surprising. The use of 'open – access' surgeries, although sometimes more difficult to manage from the health practitioners' perspective, can be more responsive to the often acute needs of families with young children, particularly in disadvantaged settings.

Nevertheless, ways of enhancing attendance for appointments that have been pursued in hospital outpatient clinics may be applicable to a community setting. For example, in one locality the proportion of Asian children who failed to attend was reduced from 50% in 1995 to 14% over a 3-year period. The intervention was multi-faceted and involved incorporating a multi-cultural calendar so as to avoid giving appointment on holy days (e.g. Fridays for Muslims) and religious festivals (such as Yom Kippur, Diwali or Chinese New Year) and also working with local communities through religious centres to explain the importance of attending for appointments. Other approaches to facilitating attendance for appointments include reminder phone calls on the day before the scheduled appointment and offering a combination of pre-booked and emergency walk-in surgeries. The newly emerging NHS walk-in centres are, we believe, likely to prove particularly popular with some ethnic minority groups.

Negotiating communication challenges

The principles of effective cross-cultural communication and importance of working with interpreters are considered in Chapters 6 and 7. However, a number of points are worth highlighting in relation to families with young children.

Although English is now the main language of communication in an increasing proportion of ethnic households, research suggests that a high proportion of women still have difficulty in conversing in English. For example, a recent survey in Walsall found that approximately one-quarter of Asian women of child-bearing age were unable to communicate in English; this compared with a figure of only 6% among Asian men. The need for health professionals to value and work with interpreting services, underpinned by knowledge of their patients and language needs, is obvious. Families with special language needs should have this information clearly marked on their computerized or manual medical records. It is also important that there is an agreed practice protocol to ensure that such information is reliably communicated to other health professionals at the time of referral.

Children as interpreters?

Although children have frequently been used as interpreters for other family members in the past, this practice is now generally discouraged on the grounds that it is unprofessional and unethical. Concerns are generally expressed on three broad fronts.

♦ A child is unlikely to be familiar with medical terminology and procedures and there is thus the risk that the translation offered is inaccurate and unreliable.

♦ There may be concerns regarding confidentiality. It is our experience that there are issues that some parents feel uncomfortable in discussing in the presence of their children, contraception and maternity care being well-known examples.

♦ Concern has been expressed in some quarters that the 'power' given to children in an interpreting role may make parents feel dependent, thus adversely affecting family dynamics.

We suggest that, whenever and wherever possible, the services of a professionally trained interpreter should be employed.

Health information

Although written resources in minority ethnic languages remain scarce, there are now a number of important initiatives. For example, many important Department of Health publications aimed at the general public are now available in a range of languages. A recently launched website (*www.mypil.com*) for both public and professionals also offers access to patient information leaflets and resources in several Asian languages, some of which aim to provide parents with information on common childhood conditions. A series of health guides with sections devoted to disorders that commonly affect young children in the languages of the main ethnic minority groupings in Britain is also available. It is hoped that such services will mushroom, both in terms of the range of languages catered for and the subject matter covered, in the near future.

Link workers and patient advocates

The roles, potentials and importance of link workers and advocates are considered in Chapter 8. Link workers seek to promote in-depth communication between patient and health care professionals, enhancing professional understanding of health needs and simultaneously facilitating patient awareness of the range of services available. The benefits that such initiatives may bring are varied and often unpredictable. For example, link workers in one area identified that the (inappropriately short) length of hospital gowns was an important barrier to mothers attending for antenatal care. In Birmingham link workers have been found to help significantly increase birth weight in 'at risk' pregnancies. An issue of particular concern to families with young children is that where such services are available they tend to be limited to certain days of the week or for a few hours each day. Although well intentioned, such services can be poorly or inappropriately advertised and therefore important sections of the target audience remain unaware of their availability.

Clinical considerations

We outline below some of the issues that we feel are particularly important for primary and community care practitioners in the context of providing routine care to children from minority ethnic communities.

Screening for haemoglobinopathies

Haemoglobin disorders form the subject of Chapter 19. Antenatal and postnatal screening for the haemoglobinopathies occurs in some parts of the UK, although the overall provision of such services is patchy. Successes have been noted, such as the prospective testing and prenatal diagnosis programme for thalassemia among London's Cypriot community which resulted in a fall in thalassemia incidence of over 40% in a 5-year period. A new national linked antenatal and neonatal screening programme for sickle cell disease and thalassemia is proposed to take effect from 2004.

Screening for HIV

The government is now committed to reducing vertical transmission of HIV, but there is concern about the higher than expected uptake of antenatal HIV screening among mothers from minority ethnic communities. This may possibly reflect a failure of antenatal staff to obtain truly informed consent from women who have difficulty in communicating in English. For example, over 95% of South Asian women (Pakistani, Bengali and Indian) in Walsall currently accept the offer of antenatal screening for HIV, compared to an uptake rate of over 65% for other mothers. It is clearly important that every effort is made to ensure that women fully comprehend the nature of the test being performed, and the possible implications of a positive test result. Link workers and advocates might facilitate this process.

Feeding and nutrition

Nutrition-related diseases in childhood may be prevented by good feeding and weaning practices. During the first few months of life, breast milk represents the optimal source of nourishment. Regional and national data show that breast-feeding is more common among South Asian mothers than white mothers. Asian mothers will also typically breast-feed for longer. It is likely that with acculturation the incidence of traditional practices such as breast-feeding in these communities will decline, unless proactive strategies are adopted to emphasize their benefits.

Iron-deficiency anaemia remains an important health concern among Bangladeshi, Hindu and Rastafarian children. Among Bangladeshis, delayed weaning and the early introduction of cow's milk within the first 12 months may largely explain this; in the other groups it seems to be due to vegetarianism. There is some preliminary research suggesting that iron-deficiency anaemia may be associated with developmental delay and breath-holding attacks, which anecdotal evidence suggests are more common among Asians. Clinicians should therefore have a relatively low threshold for investigating children presenting with either classical features of iron-deficiency anaemia or possibly related conditions such as decreased appetite, pica (ingestion of inedible material such as dirt) or breath-holding attacks. This is particularly important because treatment with iron supplementation not only improves appetite but may improve psychomotor development. The case for routine screening of children for iron-deficiency anaemia is yet to be established.

Growth monitoring

The nine-centile growth charts currently in use are based on growth patterns of European children. When interpreting growth charts of black and minority ethnic children it is important to be aware of subtle yet important differences in growth patterns that are found among ethnic and religious minorities. Thus African-Caribbean children are slightly taller on average than white children whereas the opposite is true for Asian children. Detailed study of growth patterns among Asian sub-cultures reveals that children born to Sikh mothers are heavier at birth and have better growth (height and weight) during the first 5 years of life than do offspring born to Muslim and Hindu mothers.

Pragmatic considerations dictate that it is at present not possible to develop ethnic-specific growth charts, and current guidance therefore suggests that the nine-centile chart should be routinely used for all ethnic groups, with adjustment for parental height where deemed appropriate. Importantly, the assumption that Asian children are short simply on account of their ethnicity is best avoided.

Religious circumcision

Male circumcision is important to members of the Jewish and Muslim faiths. Boys will typically be circumcised within the neonatal period and it is important that health professionals advise parents to suitably delay the procedure in infants with either prolonged jaundice or hypospadias. Jaundice increases the risks of significant haemorrhage; in cases of hypospadias the foreskin is used for reconstructive surgery. In some areas, facilities for male circumcision are now available through the National Health Service either free of charge or at a subsidized rate. Primary care organizations should consider extending the availability of such provisions to areas with high Jewish or Muslim populations. Female circumcision, discussed in Chapter 17, is important to some people of African ancestry but has been illegal in Britain since the introduction of the Female Circumcision Act in 1985.

Immunizations

Ethnic minority communities in Britain have many of the characteristics that one would associate with poor uptake of immunizations, including communication difficulties, relatively low literacy levels and an unfavourable socio-economic profile. Nevertheless, childhood immunization rates among these children are, if anything, better than those achieved in ethnic white children. Although these findings are welcome, concern has been raised that high uptake in ethnic groups may reflect a lack of awareness of the possible health risks associated with immunization (actual or perceived) among minority families. As discussed in relation to HIV screening, it is important that truly informed consent is obtained before performing any procedures.

Child abuse

Although notions of child abuse vary greatly between cultures, most, if not all, cultures unequivocally condemn the sexual or physical abuse of minors (definitions of 'minor' are also culture specific). There has to date been little research on child abuse in ethnic families. It appears that child sexual abuse is relatively uncommon in Asian households; all identified perpetrators in a Leeds-based study were male. Another salient finding to emerge from this study was that professionals were less likely to intervene in cases of suspected abuse of Asian children than for indigenous children. This perhaps reflects professional insecurity and the need for professional training in responding to diversity (see Chapter 10).

Care is needed when interpreting physical signs of physical abuse. Mongolian blue spots are common in Chinese and South Asian children, for example, and should not be confused with bruising from non-accidental injury. The degree of skin pigmentation will also affect the colour of bruising, which is typically violet or mauve in white-skinned races and a deep purple in those with darker skin.

Accidents

South Asian children in the UK are involved in twice as many pedestrian accidents as the national average, according to a recent report published by the Department of the Environment, Transport and the Regions (DETR). This is largely explained by socio-economic disadvantage and urban residence. The risk is greatest in families where parents are unfamiliar with UK traffic conditions, particularly among recent migrants. To address this problem, in 2001 the DETR launched a range of road safety advice leaflets in four Asian languages. Health visitors should be encouraged to complement this imitative with verbal advice to those families most at risk.

After all the publicity regarding the dangers linking *surma* with lead poisoning, it is now rare to see a child with this eye cosmetic. The very effective way in which health professionals joined forces with ethnic minority media services and community bodies here is, in many respects, a useful model for further health promotional initiatives.

There is no evidence to suggest that children from minority ethnic communities are at increased risk of other types of accidental injury.

Conclusion

Our better understanding of the important impact of early life events on adult health outcomes highlights the importance of focusing attention and resources on the very youngest members of minority ethnic communities. Crucial to achieving successful outcomes is that health and other professionals have a detailed understanding of the minority ethnic communities they serve. This demands the ability and willingness to work with these communities as an integral part of delivering primary and community care.

Key points

- Almost 1 in 10 children in Britain belongs to a minority ethnic group
- Health at the very beginning of life is a crucial determinant of health in later life
- Focusing attention on the health of young children is likely to reap great dividends in helping to promote health and well-being in minority ethnic communities
- Achieving improvements in the health of minority ethnic children will depend largely on the success of initiatives aimed at tackling the wider determinants of health
- Primary care organizations have a crucial role to play by taking a pro-active approach to helping promote access to equitable health care

◆ Any strategies adopted should, wherever possible, respect the indigenous traditions of the families being cared for

Acknowledgements

Aziz Sheikh is supported by a NHS R&D National Primary Care Training Fellowship.

Further information

British Medical Association. *Growing up in Britain: ensuring a health future for our children.* London: BMJ Books, 1999.

Department of Health. *Reducing health inequalities: an action report.* London: HMSO, 1999. A summary of the Department of Health's strategy for reducing health inequalities.

Dwivedi KN, Varma VP (eds). *Meeting the needs of ethnic minority children. A handbook for professionals.* London: Jessica Kingsley, 1996. Contributions from service providers discussing different strategies for working with minority ethnic families in order to deliver more equitable health care.

Gatrad AR. A completed audit to reduce hospital outpatients non-attendance rates. *Archives of Disease in Childhood* 2000; 82: 59–69.

Gould C, Rose D, Woodward P (eds). *SHAP calendar of religious festivals.* London: SHAP Working Party, 1999.

Hall DMB (ed.). *Health for all children.* Oxford: Oxford University Press, 1996.

Modood T, Berthoud R, Lakey J, Nazroo J, Smith P, Virdee S, *et al. Ethnic minorities in Britain: diversity and disadvantage.* London: Policy Studies Institute, 1997. Summary of findings from the most reliable and comprehensive survey of the demographic, socio-economic and health profile of minority ethnic communities in Britain.

Nazroo JY. *The health of Britain's ethnic minorities.* London: Policy Studies Institute, 1997.

Webb E. Meeting the needs of ethnic minority children. *Archives of Disease in Childhood* 1996: 74: 264–267.

17 Sexual health

Nicola Low

Talking about sexual health in primary care is among the most challenging of subjects. Sexual health is private, finding the right words is difficult, and the duties of confidentiality and patient care may conflict. Talking about sexual health with patients from minority ethnic groups may pose further challenges. If the patient's first language is not English, it may simply be impossible. What about negative stereotyping and inadvertent racism? In this chapter I describe what we know about the sexual health of people from minority ethnic groups in the UK. I will then discuss the sexual health consultation and management of specific problems.

Sexual health

The first ever Government strategy on sexual health in England, published in 2001, defines 'Essential elements of good sexual health [as] equitable relation-ships and sexual fulfilment with access to information and services to avoid the risk of unintended pregnancy, illness or disease'.[1] Here, I focus on the risks of sexually transmitted infections and HIV, unplanned teenage pregnancy, sexual assault and female genital mutilation.

What do we know about sexual health in minority ethnic groups?

Our knowledge of sexual health in minority ethnic groups is limited because routine data do not include ethnic group information. Unfortunately researchers also avoid this area because they fear their findings may be misused to create or perpetuate negative behavioural stereotypes.[2] This lack of accurate information is itself discriminatory, exacerbating sexual ill-health because existing stereo-types are perpetuated, important problems go unrecognized and resources cannot be appropriately targeted.

Bacterial sexually transmitted infections

Chlamydia is the most common bacterial sexually transmitted infection in the world. Gonorrhoea is less widespread, but the incidence of both infections in the United Kingdom doubled between 1995 and 2000. Genitourinary clinic data in south-east London show the highest prevalence of both infections among people from black Caribbean backgrounds (about 10 times higher than in whites) followed by those of black African origin (3–4 times higher) and similar rates in white, Asian and other ethnic groups (Figure 17.1).[3]

Similar patterns have been found in the south-east of England, Leeds, Birmingham and Coventry. Teenagers and young adults in all ethnic groups are at highest risk. In London in 1994–95, gonorrhoea and chlamydia rates in 15–19-year old women were 2.6% and 4.6% in black Caribbeans, 0.3% and 1.3% in black Africans and 0.2% and 0.4% in whites.[3] These disparities take into account age and socio-economic status but not differential utilization of genitourinary services. Young people from black ethnic groups appear to access services more than those from white or Asian groups, irrespective of diagnosis. Although this may exaggerate differences, a higher prevalence of chlamydia in black Caribbean and African women in primary care in London has also been found.[4]

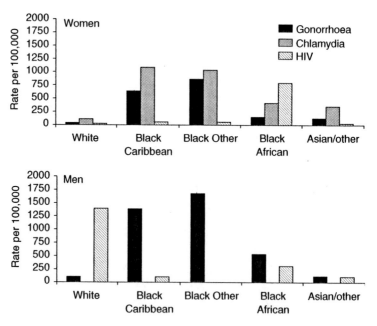

Figure 17.1 Comparison between rates of gonorrhoea, chlamydia and HIV in Lambeth, Southwark and Lewisham

Source: Data for gonorrhoea and chlamydia, 1994–95 from Low N, *et al.* 2001.[3] Figures for chlamydia in men not available. Data for HIV, 2000 from SOPHID, CDSC and London Research Company.

Viral sexually transmitted infections

The distribution of genital warts and herpes differs markedly from the patterns for bacterial infections. Genital warts, the most common sexually transmitted infection in Britain, are 2–3 times more common in the white population than in any other ethnic group. The prevalence of clinically recognized genital herpes is similar across ethnic groups, but serological studies suggest that it is more common in people from black African and Caribbean populations.

Hepatitis B is endemic in sub-Saharan (particularly West) Africa and south-east Asia where more than 90% of the population have evidence of past exposure and 10–20% may be chronic carriers in comparison with less than 1% in developed countries. Hepatitis B is sexually transmissible but is more commonly spread parenterally and vertically. Hepatitis C is rarely sexually transmitted, but parenteral spread is common in developing countries.

HIV infection

Since 1999 the most frequent route of acquisition of newly reported HIV infections has been through heterosexual sex.[6] Most homosexually acquired HIV infections are in white men (89%), but 57% of heterosexually acquired and 60% of vertically transmitted infections are in people of black African origin. Most of these adult infections were acquired in sub-Saharan Africa, mostly in Uganda and East Africa, but about 10% are thought to have been transmitted locally.[6]

The impact of more recent HIV epidemics in sub-Saharan Africa is now being seen, primarily in London where over 70% of black Africans in the UK live. In the year 2000 about 1 in 240 women who gave birth in inner London was HIV infected, compared with about 1 in 1400 in the rest of England, and most of those in London were black African.[6] The proportion of infections diagnosed before birth and thus preventable by obstetric and medical interventions is now increasing as a result of increased uptake of antenatal HIV testing.

Although absolute numbers remain small, new HIV infections reported from Asia and Latin America/Caribbean are increasing: 28% of all infections recorded as occurring in the Indian sub-continent (21/76) were reported in 2000. 30% (98/324) of all reports from Latin America/Caribbean were from Jamaica.

Unplanned and teenage pregnancy

Unplanned pregnancy is an important issue for women of all ages. I focus on teenagers because the Government has published a prevention strategy to reduce teenage pregnancy rates, which are the highest in Western Europe. Birth and termination rates differ by ethnic group, influenced strongly by migration patterns, cultural expectations and religion.

Birth rates

The Labour Force Survey shows the highest lifetime fertility rates among Pakistani and Bangladeshi women.[7] Fertility rates among Indian women are slightly higher than those of white and black Caribbean women. Teenage birth rates in all South Asian backgrounds have fallen dramatically since the 1970s, but those in white and black Caribbean teenagers have remained stable. In 1990–96 teenage birth rates were highest in Bangladeshi women (53 per 1000) and black Caribbean women (47 per 1000), similar in white women (31 per 1000) and Pakistani women (30 per 1000) and lowest in Indian women (7 per 1000).[7]

Termination of pregnancy

Ethnic group is not recorded at termination of pregnancy. However, data from the British Pregnancy Advisory Service, which carried out 27% of all abortions and 53% of NHS agency and non-NHS abortions in 1999, show that women from some minority ethnic groups were over-represented. Compared with the general population there were greater proportions of women from black Caribbean (2.1%), black African (3.1%) and black Other (0.7%) ethnic groups and lower proportions from white (88%) and Chinese (0.6%) ethnic groups. Among teenagers the pattern was similar.

Contraception

Contraceptive behaviour among South Asian women is one aspect of sexual health that has been investigated in detail. As with other ethnic groups, employment and education are the major influences on contraceptive use in women from South Asian backgrounds. Women who were not educated in Britain and not in employment are much less likely to know about contraception before their first pregnancy.

Among teenagers, qualitative studies suggest that levels of contraceptive use are similar between black Caribbean and white young women who become pregnant. Methods of contraception after delivery differ, however, with more young women from Caribbean backgrounds being fitted with intrauterine devices and more white young women being given oral contraceptives. Methods of contraception among non-pregnant teenagers from black Caribbean and black African backgrounds are similar to those from white backgrounds.

Sexual assault

In one area of south London with a specialized clinical service, data have been collected since 2000. Among women referred to the service by the police the ethnic distribution of clients was similar to that of the local population as a whole (Dr J Welch, personal communication). However, among those referring themselves, most of whom had never reported the assault to the police, women from all black ethnic groups were over-represented.

Female genital mutilation

Female genital mutilation is the excision or removal of any part of the genital organs for non-medical reasons with no obvious health benefits. Genital mutilation is illegal in this country, but up to 20 000 women in the United Kingdom are thought to have undergone it in their country of birth. Female genital mutilation is practised in 28 African countries, parts of the Middle East, Indonesia and Malaysia. The most common countries of origin for circumcised women in the UK are Eritrea, Ethiopia, Somalia and the Yemen. Specialized clinics at Northwick Park and Guy's Hospitals in London, where there are large numbers of women from countries where genital mutilation is common, offer counselling, medical and surgical help.

Key clinical issues and challenges

Most contraceptive advice takes place in primary care and most young people from black Caribbean, black African and white ethnic groups would approach their GP first if they thought they might have a sexually transmitted infection (Low N, *et al.* Unpublished report to Department of Health, 2001). The key challenge for primary care practitioners is therefore to be able to discuss sexual health issues confidently and non-judgmentally.

Taking a sexual history

The National Strategy for Sexual Health proposes an increased role for primary care in providing sexual health services. At the most basic level it suggests that all primary care teams should provide sexual history taking. Taking a sexual history is important in a range of primary care consultations, including risk assessment of women seeking contraception or termination of pregnancy, before insertion of intrauterine devices, and investigation of common presentations such as 'cystitis' or intermenstrual bleeding, which may be due to chlamydial infection.

Taking a sexual history requires confidence, sensitivity and confidentiality. It is clearly inappropriate to take a sexual history from a patient whose first language is not English and who has a family member present as an interpreter. A routine and objective approach helps avoid important omissions and reduces the chance that questions are perceived as inappropriate. The principles of good sexual history taking are:

♦ Warn the patient that you are going to ask some personal questions and reassure them about confidentiality.

♦ Ask questions in a non-pejorative way, showing that you have not made any prior assumptions about sexual lifestyle. For example, 'When did you last have sex?' and 'When did you last have sex with another partner?' rather than 'Have you had sex with anyone other than your husband?'

♦ Try not to leave out important questions because you assume that the patient is not at risk. For example, although sex before marriage is strongly censured by most religions, assuming that a young single woman from a particular religious background is not having sex may lead you to ignore symptoms due to a sexually transmitted infection or unplanned pregnancy.

A full sexual history should include questions about:

♦ duration and severity of symptoms (see Box 17.1)
♦ most recent episode of sexual intercourse:
  ■ timing (in relation to symptoms)
  ■ type and duration of relationship (regular or casual)
  ■ type of sexual intercourse (possible sites of infection)
  ■ use of condom and contraception
  ■ gender of partner (sexual orientation)
♦ details of previous sexual partners (these should be obtained in relation to duration of symptoms – to find out about new partners and who needs to be contact traced – but are also needed to assess risk in those without symptoms, given the burden of asymptomatic infection.)
♦ sexual intercourse abroad or with partners from other countries (risk of antibiotic resistant gonorrhoea, tropical sexually transmitted infections or HIV risk)
♦ previous sexually transmitted infections, tests for sexually transmitted infections including HIV, hepatitis B
♦ contraceptive choice and actual use (risk of unwanted pregnancy and infection)
♦ menstrual, cervical cytology and obstetric history in women
♦ drug history, including allergies, self treatment, non-prescribed drugs and injection drug use.

Detection and management of sexual health problems

As with many conditions, managing sexual health problems in primary care is facilitated by good communication with the patient and liaison with specialist

---

Box 17.1 **Possible symptoms and signs of some sexually transmitted infections (potential causes in brackets)**

- **Urethritis** (in men: chlamydia, gonorrhoea, non-specific urethritis, rarely trichomonas, genital herpes, warts)
  urethral discomfort or itching on micturition
  urethral discharge: purulent (typically gonorrhoea), mucopurulent or clear (typically non-specific urethritis including chlamydia)
- **Urethritis** (in women: chlamydia, gonorrhoea)
  urinary frequency or urethral discomfort, 'cystitis'
- **Cervicitis** (chlamydia, gonorrhoea)
  intermenstrual bleeding
  postcoital bleeding
  cervical mucopurulent discharge
- **Vaginitis** (trichomoniasis and non-sexually transmitted candida and bacterial vaginosis)
  vaginal soreness or irritation (trichomoniasis or candida)
  vaginal discharge: lumpy (typically candida), smelly, thin and homogeneous (typically bacterial vaginosis)
- **Proctitis** (gonorrhoea, chlamydia, herpes simplex, warts, rarely amoebiasis in homosexual men)
  rectal discomfort, discharge, lumps or ulceration
- **Conjunctivitis** (chlamydia, gonorrhoea)
- **Upper genital tract infection** (chlamydia, gonorrhoea, anaerobic infections)
  women (pelvic inflammatory disease): dyspareunia, lower abdominal pain, adnexal tenderness and/or mass, fever ± symptoms of cervicitis
  men (epididymo-orchitis): testicular swelling and pain, fever
- **Genital ulceration** (herpes simplex, syphilis, rarely chancroid, donovanosis, lymphogranuloma venereum)
- **Genital lumps** (genital warts, molluscum contagiosum, scabies)
- **Complicated infections**
  chlamydia: Reiter's syndrome (urethritis, seronegative arthritis, iritis)
  gonorrhoea: disseminated infection (arthritis, endocarditis, meningitis), Bartholin's cyst
  primary herpes simplex: urinary retention, constipation, radiculo-myelopathy, systemic viraemia

colleagues who can give advice on diagnosis and management. Shared care for chronic problems such as HIV infection is advisable. Clinical examination is important in the assessment of genital symptoms. Patients should be asked if they object to the gender of the practitioner examining them. For women from some religious and ethnic groups, only examination by a woman is acceptable.

Symptomatic sexually transmitted infections

Genital tract infections result in a limited number of clinical syndromes. Here I cover the most common syndromes of vaginal and urethral discharge. Knowledge of the differential diagnosis, refined by clinical examination and questions to assess risk can then guide appropriate therapy. The syndromic approach is recommended by the World Health Organization and widely used in resource-poor settings. In developed countries an initial syndromic assessment can guide immediate therapy while laboratory test results are awaited.

Vaginal discharge

Abnormal vaginal discharge is usually due to either endogenous (vaginal candidiasis and bacterial vaginosis) or sexually transmitted (trichomoniasis) vaginal infection. Subjective vaginal discharge without microbiological evidence of infection is commonly reported by women in Bangladesh and India. In India it is associated with a complex of symptoms of bodily weakness, aches, and mental stress and known as *kamjori* in Hindi and Gujerati.[8]

Vaginal discharge is actually a very insensitive and non-specific indicator of cervical infections (gonorrhoea and chlamydia), and speculum examination is required to identify clinical cervicitis and take specimens. The presence of mucopurulent cervical discharge is associated with cervical infections, but even this is present in only about 40% of cases of gonorrhoea or chlamydia. These infections are more common among women from African-Caribbean and deprived backgrounds.

The presence of additional risk markers such as young age, lack of condom use and a recent new sexual partner can increase the sensitivity of the clinical examination.[4] The combination of findings on clinical history and examination could be used to guide presumptive therapy while the results of microbiological tests are awaited. Endocervical specimens for both *Neisseria gonorrhoeae* and *Chlamydia trachomatis* should be taken if cervicitis is suspected.

Recommended antibiotics for treating gonococcal and chlamydial infections are published by the Medical Society for the Study of Venereal Diseases (www.mssvd.org.uk/CEG) and Clinical Evidence in the UK and the Centers for Disease Control in the USA (www.cdc.gov/std/treatment).

Urethral discharge

Urethritis in men usually presents as urethral discharge with dysuria or urethral itching. The absence of urgency, strangury and nocturia should help distinguish it clinically from the symptoms of urinary tract infection. For historic reasons urethritis is called either gonococcal, or non-gonococcal or non-specific. Some of the causes of non-specific urethritis are now known, the most common being

C. trachomatis. Ureaplasma urealyticum and *Mycoplasma genitalium* are increasingly recognized but are not routinely tested for since both respond to the antibiotics most commonly used against chlamydia.

Partner notification

The management of sexually transmitted infections includes the notification and treatment of sexual partners. Re-infection by an untreated sexual partner can lead to suppression of partially treated symptoms, delayed diagnosis of ascending infection and continued transmission. Partner notification by specialist health advisers in genitourinary clinics is often recommended. Effective communication between practice and clinic must, however, be in place to ensure attendance since as few as 11% of patients referred from community settings have been confirmed to attend a genitourinary clinic. Practice nurses can be trained to undertake partner notification and the effectiveness of this strategy is currently being evaluated. Ensuring patient confidentiality is essential for effective partner notification.

HIV infection

Most people with HIV infection have no symptoms or signs. Signs of early symptomatic disease include non-tender lymphadenopathy, oral candidiasis, seborrhoeic dermatitis and unexplained fever and weight loss. Some non-specific dermatological conditions in sub Saharan Africans are suggestive of HIV infection, including hyperpigmentation, straightening and thinning of the hair, and vertical pigmented lines on the nails. Some AIDS-defining illnesses are also more common among people with HIV from sub-Saharan Africa than white Europeans.[9] Tuberculosis is the most frequent co-existing infection, and HIV testing should always be offered. Cryptococcal meningitis and toxoplasma encephalitis occur more frequently in Africans with HIV. These infections may present with behavioural disturbance and be misdiagnosed as psychiatric disorders. HIV infection should be managed by a multidisciplinary team that includes specialist physicians and nurses, health advisers, primary care and mental health and obstetric specialists. Early diagnosis and treatment of HIV infection can reduce mortality by 70% and prevent mother to child transmission.

Asymptomatic sexually transmitted infections

Sexually transmitted infections are frequently asymptomatic, particularly in women. Up to 80% of chlamydia in women and 50% in men is asymptomatic, particularly in community settings. HIV infection has a long asymptomatic phase, and syphilis, genital herpes and chronic hepatitis B remain asymptomatic in many people after the primary infection.

Screening programmes, which can be population based or opportunistic, are used to detect asymptomatic infections. Antenatal screening for syphilis and HIV infection are good examples of programmes that detect disease at an early stage when intervention is beneficial. The requirement for universal antenatal HIV testing has increased detection rates, probably in part because there is no longer a fear of stigmatizing women from sub-Saharan Africa, which may have led to reluctance to offer them tests in the past.

Screening for asymptomatic chlamydia is being widely discussed at present. The increasing availability of nucleic acid amplification tests that can be used on non-invasively collected urine or vulvo-vaginal specimens has made this feasible. The effectiveness of a screening programme has not yet, however, been conclusively demonstrated. Proposals in the National Strategy for Sexual Health would involve testing women presenting for termination of pregnancy to prevent post-abortal infection and opportunistic testing of women having their first cervical smear.[1] This latter category will, however, miss those under the age of 20, who have the highest prevalence of chlamydia.

Hepatitis B carriers are almost always asymptomatic but may present with symptoms and signs of chronic liver disease. Since vaccination is highly effective, immunization against hepatitis B is recommended for certain groups including sexual and close family contacts of carriers, injecting drug users and babies born to mothers who are carriers. Universal antenatal screening for hepatitis B markers is cost-effective and has been recommended by the Department of Health because selective screening can miss some carriers. Screening of people from high prevalence countries may be warranted so that family contacts can be immunized.

Opportunities for prevention

Understanding the way in which people's cultural backgrounds influence sexual lifestyles and sexual health will help primary care practitioners give appropriate and relevant advice. Cultural and religious practices such as circumcision, vaginal douching, concurrent sexual partnerships and polygamy, and early marriage will all affect the risk of acquiring sexually transmitted infections.[2] These are in turn modified in second- and third-generation members of minority ethnic groups, among whom cultural norms may be more similar to those of the dominant white majority population in the UK than their parents and grandparents.

In the individual consultation, sexual health promotion opportunities rely on practitioners feeling confident about raising issues such as HIV testing with patients from sub-Saharan Africa, or testing for chlamydia in unmarried young women from African Caribbean and South Asian backgrounds.

As a practice, participating in community partnerships for example with African community-based organizations can raise awareness and destigmatize sexual health issues such as HIV, thus increasing condom use and voluntary testing rates. Primary care also has a role to play in interventions that improve access to sexual health services by providing settings for outreach clinics.[2]

Conclusion

Dealing with sexual health problems in people from minority ethnic groups relies greatly on following general principles of good-quality sexual health care. Understanding local ethnic patterns of distribution of sexually transmitted infections, unwanted pregnancy and the cultural influences on sexual behaviour is needed. Maintaining an awareness of risk, and its identification through sexual history taking where appropriate, is important in a range of clinical contexts in primary care.

Key points

◆ Sexual ill-health is an important cause of morbidity among people from minority ethnic groups

◆ Both research about sexual health issues and discussion of sexual health in primary care consultations with people from minority ethnic groups have been neglected because of embarrassment and fear of being thought to be racist

◆ Many sexually transmitted infections are asymptomatic so they should be considered in a range of situations including requests for contraception and termination of pregnancy

◆ Good sexual history taking and consultations with people from minority ethnic groups rely on effective communication and understanding the cultural and religious influences on presentation and perception of sexual health problems

References

1. Department of Health. *National strategy for sexual health and HIV infection*. London: The Stationery Office, 2001.
2. Fenton KA. Strategies for improving sexual health in ethnic minorities. *Current Opinion in Infectious Diseases* 2001; 14: 63–69.
3. Low N, Sterne JA, Barlow D. Inequalities in rates of gonorrhoea and chlamydia between Black ethnic groups in South East London: Cross-sectional study. *Sexually Transmitted Infections* 2001; 77: 15–20.

4. Oakeshott P, Kerry S, Hay S, Hay P. Opportunistic screening for chlamydial infection at time of cervical smear testing in general practice: prevalence study. *BMJ* 1998; 316: 351–352.

5. Holmes KK, Sparling PF, Mårdh P-A, Lemon SM, Stamm WE, Piot P *et al. Sexually Transmitted Diseases*. New York: McGraw-Hill, 1999.

6. Communicable Disease Surveillance Centre. *HIV and AIDS in the UK. An epidemiological review: 2000*. London: PHLS, 2001.

7. Berthoud, R. Teenage births to ethnic minority women. *Population Trends* 2001;104 (Summer): 12–17.

8. Makhlouf Obermeyer C (ed.). *Cultural perspectives in reproductive health*. New York: Oxford University Press, 2001.

9. Del Amo J, Petruckevitch A, Phillips AN, Johnson AM, Stephenson JM, Desmond N *et al*. Spectrum of disease in Africans with AIDS in London. *AIDS* 1996; 10: 1563–1569.

18 Cancer and palliative care

Christina Faull

Cancer is a powerful threat, to life itself and to the way we live. Treatment is exhausting. Our family and work life may be very disrupted and finances may alter. Life is never the same again. We change our priorities to think of and plan for a future. We may be faced with the certainty of death or the indefinite burden of hope.

Threat means fear, anger, denial, or fight. Mix with this misconceptions about cancer such as contagion, punishment, or guilt and the enormous extent of the need for care becomes apparent. So often there are also difficulties in finding and communicating with those people that can help us. All this is true to a lesser or greater extent, for everyone with cancer. This chapter considers the challenges of providing good cancer care for ethnically diverse communities. These include:

♦ those general to everyone with cancer[1,2]

♦ those general to working with people from different cultural and language backgrounds whatever the health issue (see the chapters in Section II of this book)

♦ those specific to ethnicity and cancer

♦ those specific to culture and or religion and cancer, cancer treatments, death and dying.

Access to information and services

There are more similarities than differences between communities in terms of how people live and deal with cancer. What makes it more difficult for people from ethnically diverse communities is inequality in getting information and services which will meet their needs for prevention, treatment, care and support. This may be because services don't exist, but frequently it is because services are inaccessible. For example, GPs may feel that people from ethnically diverse

---

Box 18.1   **A case history**

Mrs Ahmed has advanced cervical cancer. The intra-abdominal spread is causing obstruction of her bowel and a cutaneous faecal fistula. She speaks little English. She presented with incurable disease. She had not attended screening appointments. Her 19-year-old son says her main concern is for me [her GP] to write a letter to support her sister coming to the UK from Pakistan to look after her and the family of six children, their father having died 3 years before. The interpreter tells me that Mrs Ahmed is concerned about how they will cope at home, and whether they could have a special car parking place in her road. She feels dirty from the faeces. Above all, she is distraught that she will not be able to ensure good marriages for her children. The key issues for the practitioner here include:

♦ Communication: How can I make sure I really understand Mrs Ahmed's priorities, fears and needs? How can I ensure I am able to provide her with adequate information, counsel and symptom control?
♦ Religion: At a time when she needs to feel most 'clean', the faecal fistula is causing great spiritual anguish to Mrs Ahmed as it is both physically and spiritually polluting. How can I help her?
♦ Culture: Every parent would wish to be able to ensure happy marriages for their children, but the role of the parent in achieving this varies between cultures, especially if arranged marriages or dowries play a part.

Other issues on my mind:

♦ Why didn't she attend for screening? Has this ever been aired?
♦ What services will be acceptable for her and her family to have in her home?
♦ How do I get a car parking space sorted?
♦ Who do I write to about immigration issues?

communities have little grasp of the concept of hospice and the palliative care services available. This makes it difficult to engage patients with the potential benefits.[3]

We need to ask if our cancer services are accessible. Accessibility depends on high-quality information, communication, cultural sensitivity and competence, and appropriate gatekeeping and facilitation of access to services by primary care. Consider the illustration in Box 18.1.

Patterns of cancer

The epidemiology of cancer in relation to ethnicity is complex. Genetic, environmental and lifestyle factors are at play, influenced greatly by socio-economic status. The longer a migrated population lives in its new country the more it adopts the disease patterns of that new country, largely because of lifestyle changes (such as smoking and diet).

Although high-quality data is hard to come by because of poor monitoring of ethnicity (Chapter 4), it seems the overall incidence of cancer is generally lower in ethnically diverse groups than in the indigenous UK white population. The percentage of deaths from cancer is also lower (16% compared to 25%). This is due to a lower incidence of cancer, the age structure of the populations (minority ethnic populations being relatively younger and cancer being primarily a disease of the elderly) and a higher incidence of other killer diseases such as heart disease.

Incidence

◆ Cancer is the second commonest cause of death in almost all minority ethnic groups.

◆ The commonest cancers are the same as the majority population i.e. breast, lung, colorectal, prostate, leukaemia and lymphomas.

There is a decreased risk of certain cancers in particular groups. For example, colorectal cancer appears less common in African and South Asian communities (attributed to diet) and lung cancer is less common among South Asian women (less smoking). The incidence of breast cancer among South Asian and Chinese women is lower than in other women, but increases after migration. The protective effect of melanin makes melanoma rare in non-white groups.

There is an increased risk of certain cancers in certain groups. Explanations are partial or remain unclear. Such cancers include:

◆ oropharyngeal cancer in South Asians, especially from Bangladeshi communities (related to betel nut and tobacco chewing)

◆ hepatoma in South-East Asians, Middle Eastern and African people, and South Asian and Caribbean men (linked to infection with hepatitis B and C and alcohol)

◆ prostate cancer in Caribbean and West African men

◆ nasopharyngeal cancer in South-East Asians

◆ stomach cancer in South-East Asians

◆ cervical cancer in African-Caribbean women

◆ squamous oesophageal cancer in Chinese people (at least in certain areas of China; the effect of migration is unknown).

It is likely that the overall incidence of cancer among ethnic minority communities in the UK will increase in the next decades as the population ages, lifestyles change and environmental factors alter.

Outcomes

Survival

♦ Your chance of survival from cancer may be less if you are not white.

Work in the USA indicates that survival rates from cancers are lower for people from non-white ethnic groups. The reasons for this are unclear but probably relate to all of the following:

♦ later presentation with disease (patient delays, professional delays or a more aggressive disease course)
♦ differences in response to standard treatments
♦ differences in access to treatments.

Accessing treatment

There is currently very little information about variation in access to cancer treatments related to ethnicity. However, there is concern about possible inequalities because:

♦ the proportion of people from the diverse ethnic communities is lower than expected in trials of cancer treatments
♦ the proportion of people from diverse ethnic communities referred to specialist palliative care services is lower than expected.

Access to bone marrow transplants may be problematic since a donor must, among other things, be of similar ethnicity. Cultural and religious reasons may play a role in the low donor rates to the bone marrow register, especially from some Asian communities, but it appears more likely that lack of awareness is the key barrier.

Quality of life

There has been no systematic investigation, but research to date has highlighted a range of issues (see Box 18.2).

These issues appear to be similar for everyone with cancer of whatever background. However, they are less often resolved for ethnically diverse communities. For instance, there may be difficulties in obtaining:

♦ Asian or African-Caribbean wig types
♦ skilled counselling in appropriate language
♦ holistic pain control
♦ access to self-help and support groups.

Box 18.2   **Quality of life issues**

- Anxiety
- Fatigue
- Lymphoedema
- Support for family and carers
- Treatment-related hair loss
- Pain
- Financial difficulties

Issues related to the health institution

- Lack of familiar and enjoyable food (excellent discussion of this is available[4])
- Inadequate spiritual/religious support
- Lack of prayer and washing facilities for visitors
- Restriction on number of visitors

Risk factors and opportunities for health promotion

Smoking is the biggest cancer-related health issue. African-Caribbean men and women and Pakistani men have smoking levels similar to the UK average. Bangladeshi men have significantly higher rates of smoking than average. The NHS Asian tobacco helpline is a useful source of support for those trying to quit (see 'Further information'). Chewing betel nut or tobacco is a high-risk practice which is common among Bangladeshi men and women in particular.

The taboos of sex and death come together in cervical, breast and testicular cancers and hepatoma related to hepatitis B and C. Unprotected sex in non-monogamous relationships will increase exposure to the hepatitis B and C and human papilloma viruses. The latter is thought to be important in cervical cancer. Culturally sensitive and competent promotion of sexual health and self-examination is essential.

Delivering good cancer care

Although research is limited, consistent findings are that people from ethnically diverse communities want:

- more information about cancer, cancer treatments and cancer care services
- to reduce feelings of stigma, isolation and fear
- to improve open communication and awareness about their condition
- to gain greater control and choice in their care
- to receive more effective care.

Box 18.3   **Aspects of supportive and palliative cancer care**

- Nutrition
- Maintaining physical and social independence (social work, physiotherapy, occupational therapy)
- Finance
- Speech
- Prosthetics
- Counselling
- Pain control and physical symptom management
- Bereavement support (including for bereaved children)
- Relaxation and other benefits from complimentary therapies
- Self-help groups
- Psychological health
- Spiritual care

The ethos of cancer care

The broad aims of cancer care are to reduce the number of deaths from cancer and to provide a better experience for patients and carers.[1,2] Access to care, quality of care, and the results of treatment should not depend on who you are. Standards for all aspects of cancer care are defined.[5]

Supportive and palliative care

This focuses on the needs of patients, other than for treatments directed at the tumour itself, and carers. It is a holistic, patient centred and multi-disciplinary approach to cancer care (see Box 18.3). Such services must be aware of and address the needs of ethnically diverse communities.

How people may need help from practitioners

To be effective cancer prevention, treatment and care programmes will need to be sensitive to the beliefs, attitudes, values and lifestyles of the social groups at which they are aimed.

Cancer screening

This is highlighted in Chapter 9. The lower uptake of cervical and breast screening, particularly in Asian women, is a major concern. Many people just do not know about services. Information and support in an appropriate language and format can facilitate access. This includes appointment letters (ensuring to the correct address – in one study 40% of screening invitations were not received).

Questions to consider include:

♦ Will translated written material be good enough or, because of literacy issues, is verbal material essential?

♦ Is the technical language used understandable?

♦ Who will elicit concerns and answer questions?

Other barriers to screening are:

♦ acceptability: same-sex health care professionals is an issue for some

♦ concept: screening as a preventive measure is not understood by everyone.

Uptake can be improved by outreach workers and community-oriented models of health promotion (discussed in Chapter 9).

Diagnosis and communication

Practitioners being aware of symptoms and patterns of cancer is key to early diagnosis. Relevant guidance is available.[6] Ethnicity may potentially be a complicating factor, in that other diseases with similar symptoms may be commoner than cancer (e.g. weight loss indicating diabetes or tuberculosis). A high level of awareness and good clinical skills (most importantly the ability to obtain a good history) should, however, allow prompt referral and diagnosis.

Research indicates that whatever their ethnicity, culture or religion, most people wish to know their diagnosis and what to expect. This must be carefully explained to people in language they understand, using concepts they are familiar with. Important considerations include:

♦ Has the patient any questions or concerns?

♦ How can potential stigma be addressed and the person supported within their family and community?

♦ Have misconceptions been aired such as contagion, blame and or other beliefs about cancer?

Treatment

Treatment for cancer is tough. People feel more able to cope with surgery, chemotherapy and radiotherapy if they understand the purpose of it, what to expect (good and bad) and have had an informed choice. The religious and cultural influences of some people may mean that some issues arising in treatment require particularly sensitive exploration with individual patients in discussing treatment and addressing peoples' concerns. These include:

♦ hair loss

♦ colostomy

- prostheses
- practical issues such as family roles and the impact of fatigue
- sexuality
- complementary and alternative therapies.

Palliative and terminal care

The lower referral rates of patients from ethnically diverse communities to palliative care services are thought to reflect:

- lack of awareness of what can be offered and achieved
- services not being, or not perceived as, culturally competent
- the white or Christian image of many hospices
- the choice of patients to access services in hospital
- the varying cultural patterns of dealing with advanced illness
- the lack of help patients and their families may have in adjusting to a terminal diagnosis.

The way people cope with pain is very individual and has cultural and religious influences. People have very different views about the use of opiates for controlling pain. I have worked with some Buddhists who do not wish to have any medications. I have worked with other patients who are concerned that morphine may be used to kill them. Information, communication, respect and ongoing support with continuity of care are key.

The care of the dying and the rituals of death and grief are strongly influenced by culture and religion (see 'Further information'). We know that bereavement will be made easier if these things have been 'right' for a family. Awareness of cultural aspects of death and dying may help us be aware of some of the issues. However, as emphasized throughout this book, the key points are:

- All our patients are individual in their needs, so ask what the issues and concerns are for them, and facilitate discussion.
- Be prepared to take 'risks', as we would with patients of our own culture and language to explore people's thoughts, fears and wishes in the last part of their life.

CancerLink and other studies have identified that the commonly held belief by health care professionals that minority ethnic families prefer to rely on their own resources and do not need help from outside agencies can result in a lack of support for carers. This is most marked in the Chinese community.

Bereavement

To a large extent we do not know the quantity or quality of need. Many hospices provide both proactive and reactive bereavement services. However, most are not accessed by people from diverse ethnic backgrounds.

We may presume that patterns of grief are similar in all communities. Yet, clearly, religious and cultural concepts must have a strong influence on the specifics: angels, reincarnation, the role of the spouse, to name but a few. The support from family and the community will have a very important role in easing some of the difficulties of bereavement, but we must not assume that people do not need help even though they appear to have a lot of support.

Toward improving care

Awareness raising and information

Most research with minority communities indicates a lack of knowledge about cancer and cancer services, and a desire for more information. Such information can be produced and made more accessible (see above, and also 'Further information'). For example, culturally sensitive leaflets about specific cancers, diet, wigs, prostheses and death are available. Audiovisual material is effective for proactive dissemination of information and health promotion.

Role of health professionals

Health care professionals must improve their understanding of patients' needs for information and effective communication (see below) to enable choice, a sense of control and partnership in treatment and care processes. Moreover, they can improve their knowledge and utilization of the supportive and palliative care services available to patients.

The value of bilingual advocates is increasingly recognized (see Chapter 8). They may act as a bridge between communities and health services, providing information and support as well as often acting as skilled interpreters. Current initiatives relevant to palliative care include the 'CAPACITY' project in Birmingham.

Effective communication

Understanding about cancer is difficult when you speak English, but even more difficult when you don't and a member of the family has to act as an interpreter. You don't really know whether they are telling you what you need to know or what they think you should know.

It is difficult to talk frankly about your bodily functions though an interpreter, especially if it is a male member of your family. The link workers at the hospital are good, but they have to interpret for lots of illnesses. We would like

them to have special training so they know about cancer and understand all its terminology.
[member of an Asian women's cancer support group in Bradford, 2000]

How can you make the correct diagnosis if you can't get a full history? How can patients ask questions? How can they be supported adequately? To improve this, consider:

- access to advocates and interpreters (CancerBACUP is hoping to have a language line for interpretation by the end of 2002)
- training and support of interpreters in these emotionally charged consultations
- recording consultations (so they can be replayed and considered later by patient and family)
- working doubly hard at checking your patients' understanding.

Conclusion

As we improve data collection and invest in further research, the evidence with respect to ethnicity (genes, environment and culture) and cancer will unfold. We will understand more about cause and prevention, response to treatments and the best ways to provide care. What seems likely is that more similarities than differences will always be apparent. We must be careful not to increase a sense of otherness and compound people's exclusion.

We must however, admit and confront complexities and uncertainties, especially in provision of support and intercultural working. We need to increase our sensitivity in psycho-social care to the impact of social inequalities and the emotional dimensions of migration, ethnicity and culture (including racism and violence), on the experiences of the dying.

Key points

- Outcomes for patients with cancer from diverse ethnic communities are less good than for other patients:
  - seek to improve the uptake of cancer screening
  - ensure referral of patients in early stages of cancer
  - facilitate access to support services
- If you are a gatekeeper to services, you must do this equally well for all your patients
- There is a need and desire for more information about cancer and cancer services

- Ask patients what their concerns are: don't assume you know, find out and explore them
- Advocacy services appear to improve uptake and satisfaction with cancer services

References

1. *A policy framework for commissioning cancer services.* A report by the Expert Advisory Group on Cancer to the Chief Medical Officers of England and Wales. London: Department of Health, 1995.
2. Department of Health. *The NHS cancer plan.* London: The Stationary Office, 2000.
3. Karim K, Bailey M, Tunna KH. Non-white ethnicity and the provision of specialist palliative care services: factors affecting doctors referral patterns. *Palliative Medicine* 2000; 14: 471–478.
4. Gunarantum Y. Ethnicity and palliative care. In: Culley L and Dyson S (eds). *Ethnicity and nursing practice.* Basingstoke: Palgrave, 2001.
5. Department of Health. *Manual for cancer service standards.* London: The Stationery Office, 2000.
6. Department of Health. *Referral guidelines for suspected cancer.* London: The Stationery Office, 2000 (*http://www.doh.gov.uk/cancer*).

Further information

Cancer Research Campaign/Department of Health, Proceedings of the symposium on cancer and minority ethnic groups. *British Journal of Cancer* 1996; Supplement XXIX: S1–S82.

Field D, Hockey J, Small N (eds). *Death, gender and ethnicity.* London: Routledge, 1997.

Firth S. *Wider horizons: care of the dying in a multicultural society.* London: National Council for Hospice and Specialist Palliative Care Services, 2001.

Neuberger J. *Caring for dying patients of different faiths.* St Louis, MO: Mosby, 1994.

Several organizations provide support and information for people with cancer, although currently there are very few leaflets or tapes, and no helplines, in languages other than English. Some organizations use the language line for interpreting.

CancerBACUP (*http://www.cancerbacup.org.uk*): 3 Bath Place, Rivington Street, London EC2A 3JR. Tel: 020 7613 2121, Freephone 0808 800 1234.

Cancer Blackcare (*http://www.cancerblackcare.org*): 6 Dalston Lane, London E8 3AZ Tel: 020 7249 1097, E-mail: info@cancerblackcare.org.

CancerLink (*http://www.cancerlink.org*): specialize in networking self help groups. 11–21 Northdown Street, London N1 9BN Tel: 020 7840 7840, Freephone helpline 0808 808 0000.

Cancer EQuality and the Aifya Trust: Information and support for carers of people with cancer. 27/29 Vauxhall Grove, London SW8 1SY. Tel. 020 7582 0432, E-mail: ceqc@afiya-trust.org.

NHS Asian tobacco helplines:
Bengali 0800 169 0885
Gujarati 0800 169 0884
Hindi 0800 169 0883
Punjabi 0800 169 0882
Urdu 0800 169 0881

19 Haemoglobin disorders

Paramjit Gill and Bernadette Modell

The haemoglobin disorders—thalassaemias and sickle cell disorders—are recessively inherited conditions that have profound implications for individuals, families, and health services. Haemoglobin disorders occur in all ethnic groups, but they are most common among those whose origins are outside of Northern Europe. The major disorders cover a wide spectrum of clinical severity (Table 19.1).

Molecular basis

In adults, four alpha globin genes and two beta globin genes control the production of adult haemoglobin (haemoglobin A, $\alpha_2\beta_2$), and the amount of haemoglobin present in each red blood cell (Figure 19.1). A change in the normal DNA sequence of a globin gene can lead to an abnormal haemoglobin or a thalassaemia.

With abnormal haemoglobins, an altered haemoglobin is produced in normal amounts and carriers have 20–50% of the variant haemoglobin in their red cells. In thalassaemias there is a reduced amount of normal haemoglobin. Thalassaemia carriers are typically microcytic but are rarely anaemic because they produce an increased number of red cells.

Carriers of haemoglobin disorders

It is essential to distinguish between the many healthy carriers of haemoglobin disorders and the relatively few people who have a major haemoglobin disorder.

Table 19.1 The major haemoglobin disorders

Thalassaemias	Sickle cell disorders
β Thalassaemia major and intermedia	Sickle cell anaemia (haemoglobin SS)
Haemoglobin E/β thalassaemia	Haemoglobin S/C disease
α_0 Thalassaemia major (α thalassaemia hydrops fetalis)	Haemoglobin S/β thalassaemia
Haemoglobin H disease	Haemoglobin S/D disease

Source: Modell and Anionwu.[1]

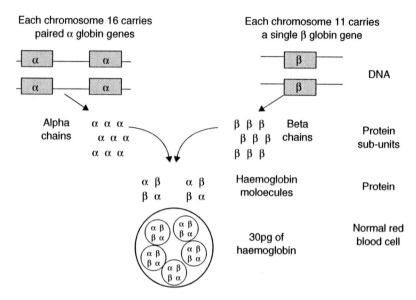

Figure 19.1 Production of adult haemoglobin

The main health implication for carriers is their genetic risk. If their partner is also a carrier, they may have a 1 in 4 risk in every pregnancy of having a child with a major disorder.

Carrier prevalence ranges from 3% to 25% among the main minority ethnic groups in the UK (see Table 19.2).[2] The corresponding birth prevalence of affected infants ranges from 0.2% to 1.6% of all children born in these groups. Up to 13% of children born in the UK are in groups at risk for haemoglobin disorders, and about 0.42/1000 of conceptions have a major haemoglobin disorder. Thus, despite their uneven distribution, average prevalence is similar to cystic fibrosis (0.45/1000 conceptions).

Major haemoglobin disorders

In the UK, there are estimated to be more than 800 patients with a major beta thalassaemia (largely from South Asian/Asian/Mediterranean backgrounds) and more than 6000 with sickle cell disorder (largely from African-Caribbean communities).[1]

Thalassaemias

In the major thalassaemias, inability to produce normal haemoglobin leads to ineffective erythropoiesis and profound anaemia.

Table 19.2 Estimated prevalence of carriers of haemoglobin disorders, affected births and at-risk pregnancies in ethnic minority groups in the UK

Ethnic group	Per cent of the population carriers					Rate per 1000 pregnancies		
	AS	AC	β thalassaemia	α_0 thalassaemia	Hb E	Total carriers	At-risk pregnancies	Affected fetuses
White	11	4	0.1	+	+	16	0.001	0.00025
Black Caribbean	22	3	0.9	+		25	22.4	5.6
Black African	11	4	1.0		+	16	62.4	15.6
Black other			0.9	+	+		22.4	5.6
Indian	+		4.3		+	4.3	1.85	0.46
Pakistani	+		4.5		+	4.5	4.0	1.0
Bangladeshi			2.8		4.5	7.3	3.3	0.826
Chinese			3.0	5.0	+	8.0	3.4	0.85
Other Asian	+	+	3.0			3.0	0.9	0.225
Other other	5		1.0	+		6.0	4.16	1.04
Cypriot	0.5–1		16.0	1.5		17.5	17.32	4.33
Italian	+		4.0			4.0	0.8	0.2

AC, haemoglobin C trait; AS, sickle cell trait; Hb E, haemoglobin E trait; SCD, sickle cell disorder.

Alpha thalassaemia major

Here the fetus develops severe anaemia, leading to heart failure and death before or immediately after birth. Maternal risks include pre-eclampsia or eclampsia, obstructed delivery, and pre- and postpartum haemorrhage.

Beta thalassaemia major

This is characterized by severe anaemia, usually diagnosed before 1 year of age. Treatment consists of monthly blood transfusions to maintain a normal haemoglobin level, splenectomy, and nightly subcutaneous infusion of the iron-chelating agent desferrioxamine to control transfusional iron overload.

Most patients who manage this burdensome treatment complete their education, work and find a partner, and are expected to live at least until their mid-forties.[3] However, conventional iron chelation therapy is intolerable for many adolescents and young adults. Up to 50% of patients still die in early adult life from the cardiac complications of iron overload.

Recent, more acceptable regimens include disposable desferrioxamine infusors and oral iron chelation. Bone marrow transplantation is an option for the 25% of young patients who have a fully compatible related donor, offering potential cure.

Although specialist care predominates, primary care teams need to be particularly aware of the risk of overwhelming infection in splenectomized patients, and of *Yersinia* (and possibly *Klebsiella*) infection in patients on desferrioxamine, and refer patients urgently if suspected.

Sickle cell disorders

In sickle cell disorders the red blood cells tend to change from their normal round shape to a rigid sickle shape. If sickled cells become trapped in blood vessels, this prevents oxygen from reaching the tissues and causes severe pain and tissue damage. Factors that can precipitate sickling include hypoxia, dehydration, sudden changes in temperature, acidosis, infection or strenuous exertion.

Clinical features

Sickle cell disorders cause anaemia, an increased risk of serious infection, and painful crises. An outstanding characteristic is unpredictability: some patients have few problems, but others become permanently disabled. The frequency and severity of complications can vary markedly. Life-threatening complications include overwhelming infection, acute chest syndrome, stroke, and (in children) splenic or hepatic sequestration of red cells. There is a risk of sudden death, but median survival is now 42 years in men and 48 years in women.[3]

Symptoms often start at 3–6 months of age, typically with 'hand–foot syndrome' – a painful swollen wrist or ankle due to small infarctions in the epiphyses of the long bones. Most affected children become functionally asplenic (sickling impedes splenic circulation), and most affected adults are asplenic (due to splenic infarction).

Management

Primary care teams need to be alert to the high prevalence of sickle cell disorders in black minority ethnic groups. These disorders may be diagnosed for the first time at any age. Neonatal screening is practised in an increasing number of areas. The NHS haemoglobinopathy screening programme has recently agreed that there should be universal neonatal screening for sickle cell disorders. This has implications for primary care, as it will be essential to track all affected children and ensure they are appropriately followed at an expert centre: much of this responsibility must fall to GPs. All children should be referred to a specialist centres for management (see below). However, if these are distant some tasks may fall to the primary care team. The most important components of management include:

- early, preferably neonatal diagnosis, enabling early protective measures
- education of parents about risks and their prevention, detection and management (e.g. infections and splenic sequestration crises)
- prophylactic penicillin from 4 months of age to reduce pneumoccocal and other infections (there is debate on the appropriate age to stop)
- immunization against *Pneumococcus* and *Haemophilus.*
- supportive therapies and treatment of acute crises with fluid therapy, pain relief, and blood transfusion; bone marrow transplantation helps some
- psychological support and counselling to facilitate coping. the unpredictable and very painful nature of complications creates severe stress for patients and families
- referral to relevant local support associations (see 'Further information').

Carrier screening

The 'haemoglobinopathy screen' combines measurement of the red cell indices (for microcytosis typical of thalassaemias) and electrophoresis for abnormal haemoglobins. The sensitivity and specificity of this blood test are extremely high.

Rationale

The objective of screening is to identify carriers and carrier couples and enable them to make an informed choice about prenatal diagnosis and selective abortion of affected fetuses. The introduction of DNA diagnostic methods has made a fetal diagnosis possible by 10–11 weeks gestation, increasing the acceptability of prenatal diagnosis to women of any ethnic group.

When performed as recommended, carrier screening detects over 96% of couples at risk of having children with a haemoglobin disorder.[3] The high level of genetic risk associated with carrier status is not generally appreciated: carriers with a partner from their own ethnic group have a 3–25% risk of forming an at-risk couple, depending on carrier prevalence in that particular group.

Consanguineous marriage

A consanguineous marriage is a marriage between close relatives, usually second cousins or closer. There is a high prevalence of such marriages in couples of Pakistani, Bangladeshi or Middle Eastern origin. For example, over 70% of British Pakistanis marry a relative, and 55% a first cousin.[4] Under these circumstances, when a pregnant thalassaemia carrier is detected there is a 16% chance that her partner is also a carrier, and a 4% risk of an affected fetus.

Although increasing a couple's risk of having children with a recessively inherited disorder, a consanguineous kinship pattern has important social advantages, particularly for women in some societies. The preference for marriage to a relative is not restricted to Muslim communities but is found in many cultures throughout the world.

Experience of carrier screening

Screening is a multiprofessional activity involving different health workers, crossing administrative boundaries. Effective screening relies on a clear local policy. It is then possible to identify and counsel practically all at-risk couples in their first pregnancy. Sadly, with present antenatal booking practice this is rarely achieved before the second trimester. First-trimester prenatal diagnosis should be offered in all subsequent pregnancies.

In one national audit the utilization of prenatal diagnosis for thalassaemia was shown to vary (50–90%), being higher at expert centres. Most affected conceptions to Cypriot parents ended in termination of pregnancy, whereas most to parents of Pakistani origin ended in an affected live-birth.[4] The difference was widely interpreted to mean that Muslim couples decline prenatal diagnosis because of religious objections to abortion. However, a confidential enquiry found the main reason was inequality of access and service delivery for the families concerned.[5]

Sickle cell and thalassaemia counselling centres are sited in areas of high prevalence, mostly in inner-city areas. They have tended to rely on committed individuals. To date appropriate service and professional development has been patchy, compounded by lack of interpreting services and bilingual counsellors. The introduction of a national screening policy, currently in development, should now help. Primary care trusts must play a crucial role in service planning and provision. A model specification for services for haemoglobin disorders is available.[3]

Primary care role in genetic risk detection and counselling

Information and screening for haemoglobin disorders should be provided in primary care, either before pregnancy or as soon as a pregnancy is notified.

Primary care professionals should be able to provide basic advice on genetic reproductive risk for their practice population. Such advice should be part of family planning, early pregnancy care, and sexual health and community initiatives. This applies whether the individual or couple are of Northern European origin, or come from an ethnic group where haemoglobin disorders or cousin marriage are common. The following recommendations apply not just for haemoglobin disorders but all other inherited disorders.

Primary care for reproductive genetic risk

Provide correct information on common genetic risks.

◆ Take a basic genetic family history.

◆ Provide pre-pregnancy or early pregnancy advice (re diet, smoking, alcohol, and folate supplementation).

◆ Carrier testing should be offered for common inherited disorders (haemoglobin disorders, cystic fibrosis, Tay–Sachs disease, as appropriate).

◆ For haemoglobin disorders, carriers detected by screening should be informed of their risk and arrangements made for rapid testing of the partner. Carrier couples should be referred urgently for expert genetic counselling and the offer of prenatal diagnosis. Standardized, clear and simple patient information materials are available at *www.chime.ucl.ac.uk/APoGI/*. They are designed to be printed out and given to patients, and a copy is kept in the notes.

If a child or adult with an inherited disorder is registered with the practice

◆ Ensure parents receive (or have received) expert genetic counselling, including clear information on the recurrence risk, feasibility of carrier testing and prenatal diagnosis for the disorder. Genetic counselling should be in the parents' preferred language.

- When the mother is pregnant, refer her in the first trimester of pregnancy, with clear information on genetic risk, directly to the appropriate specialist service (medical genetics, fetal medicine, disease-specific service).

- Consider the indications for carrier testing and genetic counselling for relatives, for example brothers and sisters (50% of the first-degree relatives of a carrier are also carriers).

- Assist specialist services in conducting family studies. Help to follow up relatives registered with the practice in order to offer genetic counselling and carrier testing when feasible.

For people who are considering marrying, or are already married to a relative

- Provide correct information about the genetic implications of cousin marriage.
- Enquire carefully into the genetic family history.
- When there is no evidence of an inherited disorder in the extended family, inform the couple of the increased genetic risk associated with cousin marriage. Offer available carrier tests for common recessive disorders. Give general pre-pregnancy advice. Tell the couple to report a pregnancy as early as possible, and refer for obstetric consultation in the first trimester of pregnancy.

- When there may be an inherited disorder in the extended family, seek more details and refer the couple to the appropriate specialist service for further investigations.

- When there is a known inherited disorder in the extended family, contact the relevant specialist service to enquire whether carrier testing and prenatal diagnosis are feasible. If they are, ensure that they are offered to the couple in the context of expert genetic counselling and specialist services, in the woman's preferred language, with referral in the first trimester. Explain that any marriage within their extended families could be at risk for the same disorder, providing appropriate information and referral for counselling.

Finally, expert counselling may be most effectively provided in primary care premises, or at the home of a family member. Some necessary specialist services, including access to expert genetic counselling in the family's preferred language, are not widely available in the UK. They will only become more available if primary care teams demonstrate demand by appropriately referring couples and families who need the service.

Key points

- Sickle cell disorders and the thalassaemias are common
- Prevalence varies between ethnic groups

♦ Life expectancy is increasing

♦ Referral for pre- and postconception counselling is crucial

♦ Primary care, expert centres and the voluntary sector all have important roles.

References

1. Modell B, Anionwu A. In: *Ethnicity and health: reviews of literature and guidance for purchasers in the areas of cardiovascular, mental health and haemoglobinopathies.* Report No 5, NHS Centre for Reviews and Dissemination/Social Policy Research Unit. CRD: York University, 1996.
2. Health Education Authority. *Sickle cell and thalassaemia: achieving health gain guidance for commissioners and providers.* London: HEA, 1998.
3. Zeuner D, Ades AE, Karnon J, Brown J, Dezateux C, Anionwu EN. *Antenatal and neonatal haemoglobinopathy screening in the UK: review and economic analysis.* Leeds: The Health Technology Assessment Panel, NHS Executive, 1999.
4. Modell B, Petrou M, Layton M, Varnavides L, Slater C, Ward RHT, Rodeck C, Nicolaides K, Gibbons S, Old J. Audit of prenatal diagnosis for haemoglobin disorders in the United Kingdom: the first 20 years. *BMJ* 1997; 315: 779–784.
5. Modell B, Harris R, Lane B, Khan M, Darlison M, Petrou M, Old J, Layton M, Varnavides L. Informed choice in genetic screening for thalassaemia during pregnancy: audit from a national confidential enquiry. *BMJ* 2000; 320: 325.

Further information

Weatherall DJ. Disorders of the blood. In: Weatherall DJ, Ledingham JGG, Warrell DA (eds). *Oxford Textbook of Medicine*, 3rd edn. Oxford: Oxford University Press, 1996. A comprehensive account of the pathophysiology and management of the haemoglobinopathies.

Streetly A, Maxwell K, Mejia A. *Sickle cell disorders in Greater London: a needs assessment of screening and care services.* The Fair Shares for London report 1997. (Available from The Directorate of Public Health, Bexley and Greenwich Health Authority, 221 Erith Rd Bexleyheath, Kent DA7 6HZ. Also from OSCAR Trust, 5 Lauderdale House, Gosling Way, London SW9 6JS.) Provides valuable information for planning sickle cell services.

Modell M, Wonke B, Anionwu E, Khan M, Tai SS, Lloyd M, Modell B. A multidisciplinary approach for improving services in primary care: randomised controlled trial of screening for haemoglobin disorders. *BMJ* 1998; 317: 788–791. Gives a model of increasing screening uptake within a locality.

NHS Haemoglobinopathy Screening Programme (*http://www-phm.umds.ac.uk/haemscreening*)

Sickle Cell Society (*http://www.sicklecellsociety.org*)

UK Thalassaemia Society (*http://www.ukts.org*)

20 Care of refugees and asylum seekers

Angela Burnett

> When you're a refugee your life is never complete. There is always part of your
> life that is missing, and that part is home.
> [Adil, a child refugee from Somalia]

Almost 1 person in 100 in the world is displaced by conflict or civil unrest.
There are over 21 million refugees worldwide, with a further 25 million people
displaced within their own countries. The vast majority of refugees remain in
countries neighbouring their own.

Asylum applications in the UK numbered 80 315 in 2000, dropped to 71 365 in
2001 and rose to 85 865 in 2002.[1] In 2000 the UK ranked 9th among EU countries and 78th in the world in terms of asylum seekers per head of population,
with 1.7 asylum seekers/1000 population.[2] This compares with the largest host
countries, Armenia, Guinea and the Federal Republic of Yugoslavia, which host
80, 59 and 46 refugees per 1000 national population respectively.[3]

Most of those seeking asylum in the UK come from countries in conflict,
many of which are fuelled by arms sold by richer countries. During 2002 the top
five countries from which asylum seekers arriving in the UK originated were
Afghanistan, Iraq, Zimbabwe, Somalia and China.[1]

Some people have been detained and tortured in their own countries because
of political or religious beliefs and activities. For others their gender, sexual
orientation, social or ethnic identity may have led to their persecution. Some are
forced to leave because of environmental disasters or engineering projects.
Others migrate due to poverty, as disparities widen between rich and poor
people, both between and within countries.

Refugees are not a homogenous group. They have different experiences and
expectations of life, health and health care. This chapter outlines the range of
health issues that may be faced by refugees and asylum seekers, and how health
and other professionals can respond to these. The term refugee may include asylum seekers and people at all stages of the asylum process. Most of those seeking
asylum in the UK are single men aged under 40, although worldwide most

refugees are women. Many refugee families are without one parent, and some children are alone.

Refugee status

In order to be recognized as a refugee, an asylum seeker must fulfil the terms of the 1951 Geneva Convention and demonstrate that:

> ...owing to a well founded fear of being persecuted for reasons of race, religion, nationality, membership of a particular social group or political opinion is outside the country of his nationality and is unable, or owing to such fear, is unwilling to avail himself of the protection of that country...
> [United Nations 1951 Convention relating to the Status of Refugees—the Geneva Convention]

The various definitions of refugee status are explained in Box 20.1. All of these groups have the full entitlement to NHS treatment available to all legal residents in Britain, and do not have to pay fees or otherwise prove their rights.

Recently arrived asylum seekers, without access to accommodation themselves, are the responsibility of the Home Office National Asylum Support Service (NASS) and are dispersed throughout the UK. They are not allowed to

---

Box 20.1   Definitions of refugee status

Asylum seeker	A person who has submitted an application for protection under the Geneva Convention and is waiting for the claim to be decided by the Home Office
Refugee status	Accepted as a refugee under the Geneva Convention and granted Indefinite Leave to Remain (ILR)—permanent residence in the UK. Eligible for family reunion (one spouse and any child of that marriage under the age of 18)
Exceptional Leave to Enter or Remain (ELE or ELR)	The Home Office accepts there are strong reasons why the person should not return to the country of origin. ELR grants the right to stay in the UK for 4 years. The person is expected to return if the home country situation improves. Ineligible for family reunion.
Refusal	The person's application for refugee status is rejected but there is a right of appeal, within strict time limits
Family reunion	Spouse and children under the age of 18 of a person who is given refugee status. They are given Indefinite Leave to Remain (ILR)—permanent residence in the UK.

work, and are entitled to 70% of income support. It is currently planned to issue asylum seekers with smart cards, to house them in induction and accommodation centres, and to explore taking refugees nominated by the United Nations directly.

Detention

Asylum seekers, including children, are increasingly being detained either in detention centres or in prisons, although they are not charged with any crime. People have no idea how long they will be detained. The effect of detention on mental health is significant, compounding feelings of isolation, depression and anxiety, particularly for those who have previously experienced detention or torture in their own country.

Becoming a refugee

Refugees have experienced many losses including separation from family, bereavement, home, friends, money, job and identity, role, status, dignity and hope. Those making the often arduous and dangerous journey into exile have courage, resourcefulness and resilience. After the initial relief however, frustration and disillusionment may ensue. Multiple losses, the absence of usual supports, racism, discrimination, isolation, diminished self-esteem, and increasing dependence and poverty may all compromise health.

It is important to enable refugees to develop independence, acquire language, gain education and employment. Integration requires support from the local community. But available housing for asylum seekers is often in deprived areas, which are already struggling for resources. Misinformation and racism targeting refugees must be challenged and prevented, and services improved for the whole community.

Improving access to health care

Free entitlement and GP registration

All asylum seekers and refugees are freely entitled to all NHS care. Those on low income should apply with an HC1 form for a certificate, giving free prescriptions, dental treatment, optician services and travel costs to hospital (available from the Department of Health response line, Tel: 0870 155 5455). Certificates are only valid for 6 months, after which a new application must be made.

Registering a new patient in general practice provides an important opportunity to establish the health needs, language needs, and social circumstances. However, many issues only become apparent later.

Permanent, rather than temporary, registration with a GP is preferable, facilitating a health check, screening, health promotion, immunizations, continuity of care and access to existing records. Patient-held records may be useful for asylum seekers, who are frequently moved around, but cramped living conditions and lack of privacy may make confidentiality difficult to maintain.

Communication and interpreting

Bilingual workers are crucial in providing services to refugees, facilitating communication and understanding of cultural background (see Chapters 7 and 8). Specific details are needed, both of language spoken (e.g. Arabic spoken in Sudan is different from Arabic spoken in Algeria) and also the language with which a person feels comfortable (e.g. many Kosovar Albanians can speak Serbo-Croat, but may not feel comfortable doing so).

Continuity of interpreter can enhance development of trust between patient, interpreter and health worker. However, exiled communities may reflect conflict in the home country, and interpreters may be viewed with suspicion. Ground rules of confidentiality must be established and made clear to both patient and interpreter.

Information on services and health promotion

Translated written information can be useful, but other methods will be more effective for those who are not literate. Oral traditions are strong among many refugee communities (e.g. Somali) and story telling, video, and audiotapes have been used to disseminate information. Health advocates, peer educators, refugee community organizations and outreach work can increase awareness about health issues, health promotion and how to access health services.

Working with communities

Refugee communities and organizations should play a key role in planning of services. It is particularly important to develop links with refugee community organizations and support them to build their capacity to provide advocacy, orientation, social support networks, information in people's own language and a connection with their own culture. Religious groups and communities can provide much emotional and practical support, as well as social contact.

The skills and experience of refugees are currently under-realized. For example, they include doctors, nurses, and other health workers, keen to get back to work and address the current skills shortage. The process of achieving this is slowly being addressed.[4]

Support for health workers

Working with refugees is rewarding but challenging. It is important not to set up unrealistic expectations and not to 'rescue' people—encourage independence, not dependence. Listening to people's accounts of their experiences may expose health workers (including administrative staff) to much distress and support may be needed.

Facing multiple problems, it is easy to feel isolated and impotent or to feel pressured to solve them, while lacking the information, skills or time to do so. Supportive partnerships between statutory and voluntary sectors, and between different disciplines can improve effectiveness and reduce isolation.

Health problems

As with anybody, the health of a refugee is affected by overlapping physical, psychological and environmental factors requiring a holistic approach. Some significant issues are outlined below.

Nutrition

Limited finance, language difficulties and lack of choice may result in a restricted diet, and culturally familiar and acceptable food may not be attainable in many dispersal areas. Asylum seekers may have previously experienced long-term food shortages, resulting in malnutrition, rickets, scurvy and thiamine deficiency.

Common conditions

As with the majority population, acute problems such as respiratory illness, musculoskeletal complaints, gastrointestinal symptoms and dental conditions are common. Fungal skin infections and scabies, often related to poor conditions during travel or in temporary accommodation, may arise. Parasitic disease, gastroenteritis (usually due to common pathogens posing little risk to public health) and more rarely, cholera, bacillary dysentery and typhoid, can occur.

The importance of addressing major chronic disease such as diabetes, hypertension, coronary heart disease and haemoglobinopathies are highlighted elsewhere in this book.

Communicable disease

Although asylum seekers should not be viewed as prominent vectors of infection, those coming from areas where infectious diseases are prevalent may carry heightened risk of infection. New arrivals need access to TB screening using past history, questions concerning symptoms and Heaf test and chest X-ray if indicated. Hepatitis B, malaria, hepatitis A and meningitis may be more common depending on country of origin and established risk factors. People may not have had immunizations listed for their country (see 'Further information'). Children should be fitted into the UK national programme, depending on their age.

HIV and AIDS

Some may have been at risk of HIV: through rape, unprotected sex in situations of high prevalence, paid sex (which refugee women may be forced to use in order to survive), through blood transfusion, contaminated needles, intravenous drug use or mother-to-child transmission.

It is inappropriate to screen everyone. Time and sensitive discussion is needed, and those at risk should be offered information, and voluntary testing for HIV and other sexually transmitted infections. People may mistrust interpreters, or fear that a positive HIV test could lead to deportation. Confidentiality needs to be emphasized.

Those who are HIV positive have full entitlement to treatment. Access to specialist legal advice is also important, as they may have compassionate grounds to remain. HIV-positive asylum seekers, who are advised not to breast-feed, recently achieved entitlement to milk tokens after a legal challenge.

Emotional well-being and mental health

Physical expressions of distress

As with anybody, stress may manifest as physical symptoms posing challenges for patient and practitioner. Take such complaints seriously, and avoid giving reassurances that they will 'go away with time'. Counselling or complementary therapies may be helpful.

Anxiety and depression

Symptoms of anxiety, depression, guilt and shame and poor sleep patterns are very common. People may have problems with memory, concentration and disorientation, which hinder learning, including that of language. These may be a result of past experiences, including conflict and torture, recent stay in a detention centre (although not charged with any crime), or people's current situation. Social isolation and poverty have a compounding effect, as do hostility and racism. Uncertainty and the fear of being sent home dominate the lives of asylum seekers. The risk of suicide and attempted suicide may rise if a person's asylum application is refused.

Care of psychological health

Diagnosis and treatment is made more complex as psychological health is particularly culture bound, compounded by difficulties with language and communication. Rather than making an initial diagnosis, it may be preferable to maintain an open mind during a long period of assessment (see Chapter 14 for further discussion of mental health and diversity).

Supportive listening, reducing isolation and dependence, having suitable accommodation, and being occupied with education or work can do much to relieve sadness and anxiety. Given the stigma mental ill-health carries, offering services in the community is likely to be more acceptable, with access to bilingual health workers or interpreters, focusing on cultural strengths and existing natural support systems. Depression among refugees is closely linked with poor social support.[5]

Counselling

Counselling may be an unfamiliar concept for some people, who are more accustomed to discussing problems with family and community rather than with a stranger and may be concerned about confidentiality. Some members of refugee communities are trained in counselling skills, which can be used in culturally appropriate ways.

Groups may offer support and reduce isolation – these may be primarily therapeutic, or more social and practical in nature. Many refugees wish to tell their story and find the process of testimony itself to be therapeutic, but it should not be assumed that people must do this in order to recover, and some find talking about their experiences extremely distressing and unhelpful.

Torture and organized violence

Torture is '... the intentional infliction of severe pain or suffering, whether physical or mental, upon a person in the custody or under the control of the accused' (Article 7.2 (e) (excerpt) of the Rome Statute of the International Criminal Court 1998).

Estimates of the proportion of asylum seekers who have been tortured or experienced organized violence vary from 5% to 30%.[6] Many do not initially admit to their experiences. This may be through shame or unwillingness to disclose sensitive information, for example sexual violation. Some methods of torture are commonly experienced, such as beating, kicking and slapping.

The effects of torture are an accumulation of physical violence and conditions of detention (unhygienic cells, inadequate diet), and the psychological consequences of one's own and witnessing others' experiences. A survivor of torture may have a preoccupation that his or her body has been irreparably damaged, leading to repeated consultations.

Physical effects of torture and trauma

Inadequately treated injuries from torture, landmines or shrapnel can result in malunited fractures, osteomyelitis, amputation, neuropathies and muscle weakness with permanent disability. Wounds and burns may be infected and keloid scars distressing. Pain, weakness and other non-specific symptoms are common, and may be helped by physiotherapy, non-steroidal analgesics, massage, relaxation and techniques to manage symptoms.

Post-concussion syndromes may present with problems of memory and concentration, but these symptoms can also be stress-related. Slapping around the ears is common during interrogations, causing tympanic perforation and otitis media. People who have been detained in darkness for long periods often complain of soreness and watering of the eyes in bright light. Recognition of the long-term effects of chemical warfare is increasing (see 'Further information').

Psychological effects of torture and organized violence

Common experiences after trauma included distressing dreams, poor sleep, recurrent vivid memories, headaches, irritability, chest or abdominal discomfort, muscle pains and feeling weak or easily tired, low mood and frequent crying. It is important to relieve symptoms, but remember that these are common responses and do not necessarily indicate mental illness.

Helpful responses

- Listen.
- Don't expect to do too much in one session.
- Have contact with and get support from other workers.
- Remember cultural differences and attitudes to health, including religious and spiritual influences.[7]

Consider carefully before pathologizing what may be natural expressions of grief and distress concerning highly abnormal experiences. The diagnosis of post-traumatic stress disorder (PTSD) should be used cautiously, and with regard to different cultural and social settings.

Specialist help may be needed where there are, for example, suicidal ideas or plans, social withdrawal and self-neglect, consistent failure to function properly with daily tasks or behaviour or talk that is abnormal or strange within the person's own culture.

Sexual and domestic violence

Many women and some men are survivors of sexual violence and rape. In many cultures these are taboo, and survivors may feel deep shame and very uncomfortable discussing their experiences.

Women who are refugees are particularly vulnerable to domestic violence, as they may lack family and community support. They may fear being alone more than they fear a violent relationship. Their partner's violent behaviour may be tolerated because of the violence that he has experienced. Women whose partner is the main applicant may lose their access to asylum if they separate and will need independent legal advice.

Needs of family members

Displacement is difficult for all, but women are often most affected. Their needs may not be identified, especially in cultures where the man is usually the spokesperson. Most asylum seekers are young men, unused to living alone, who are bored and frustrated. Within families, women may find it easier to obtain work and this may distort family relationships. Many people will have been forced to leave family behind, and may not know their whereabouts (see 'Further information').

Older people may have more difficulty in adjusting, and in particular find it harder to acquire English, so they may be very isolated. Asylum seekers with a disability may not have access to support from social services, and have great difficulties with inappropriate housing.[8] Most carers are women and they are generally unsupported and isolated.

Children

Children may be living within a fragmented family, or may be unaccompanied. They may have experienced or witnessed violence, or have been forced to commit violent acts themselves as child soldiers. Children may have developmental inconsistencies—at home they may take on responsibility, often because they speak more English than their parents, but they may be immature in other situations such as school. They may experience anxiety, aggression, poor concentration, nightmares, withdrawal, and regressive behaviour such as bedwetting or hyperactivity.

Very few children need psychiatric treatment. Support needs to be multifaceted, providing as normal a life as possible, a sense of security, promoting education and self-esteem and supporting parents. School is important but be aware of the possibility of bullying and racism –'asylum seeker' is a regular playground taunt. Refugee support teachers can provide help to refugee children and their families.

Unaccompanied children are especially isolated and vulnerable, and require ongoing contact with social services, needs assessment and a care plan, which should be regularly monitored (see 'Further information').

Conclusion

Refugees should be respected and valued as an asset to our communities. Rather than draining countries' resources, migrants have been shown overall to contribute to economies.

Health workers and systems should individualize care, in order to help people to rebuild their lives. This needs to be integrated with the building of links with community organizations, facilitating education, employment and social support networks.

> How you are with the one to whom you owe nothing, that is a grave test and not only as an index of our tragic past. I always think that the real offenders at the half way mark of the century were the bystanders, all those people who let things happen because it didn't affect them directly. I believe that the line our society will take in this matter on how you are to people to whom you owe nothing is a signal. It is the critical signal that we give to our young and I hope and pray that it is a test we shall not fail.
> [Rabbi Hugo Gryn, Holocaust survivor]

Key points

- The UK, as a signatory to the 1951 Geneva Convention, is committed to consider asylum applications from those fleeing from persecution
- Most asylum seekers are from countries that are in conflict
- Asylum seekers and refugees are entitled to full NHS care – services for them should be of similar range and quality to those of the local community
- Access to interpreting services is crucial for all staff if language is not shared
- Cultural factors should be considered when assessing health, particularly for psychological health
- Symptoms of psychological distress are common. Carefully consider before pathologizing what may be natural responses to highly abnormal situations
- Much can be done by health workers to alleviate the physical and psychological effects of torture
- Children may have experienced torture themselves or have witnessed others being tortured. Support for them needs to be multifaceted. Unaccompanied minors are particularly vulnerable

References

1. Home Office. Statistics (http://www.homeoffice.gov.uk/).
2. Refugee Council (*http://www.refugeecouncil.org.uk/news/myths/*).
3. Home Office. *Secure borders, safe haven, integration with diversity in modern Britain*. White Paper on Immigration and Asylum, 2002 (Figures from United Nations High Commissioner for Refugees, *www.unhcr.ch/statist*).
4. Cheeroth S, Goraya A. Refugee doctors. *BMJ* 2000; 321: 2–7.
5. Gorst-Unsworth C, Goldenberg E. Psychological sequelae of torture and organised violence suffered by refugees from Iraq. Trauma related factors compared to social factors in exile. *British Journal of Psychiatry* 1998; 172: 90–94.

6. Burnett A, Peel M. The health of survivors of torture and organised violence. *BMJ* 2001; 322: 606–609.
7. Shackman J, Gorst-Unsworth C, Summerfield D. *Common experiences after trauma.* London: Medical Foundation for the Care of Victims of Torture, 1996.
8. Roberts K, Harris J. Disabled people in refugee and asylum seeking communities. Bristol: The Policy Press, 2002.

Further information

Burnett A, Fassil Y. *Meeting the health needs of refugees and asylum seekers in the UK: an information and resource pack for health workers.* London: Directorate for Health and Social Care, 2002. Available online at *http://www.london.nhs.uk/newsmedia/publications/Asylum_Refugee.pdf* (This includes an extensive list of useful resources and further contacts).

Bracken P, Petty C (eds). *Rethinking the trauma of war.* London: Save the Children Fund, 1998.

Burnett A, Peel M. What brings asylum seekers to the United Kingdom? *BMJ* 2001; 322: 485–488.

Burnett A, Peel M. The health needs of asylum seekers and refugees *BMJ* 2001; 322: 544–547.

Harris K, Maxwell C. A needs assessment in a refugee mental health project in North-East London; extending the counselling model to community support. *Medicine, Conflict and Survival* 2000; 16: 201–215.

Sidell F, Hurst C. Long-term health effects of nerve agents and mustard. In: *Medical aspects of chemical and biological warfare*, Washington, DC: Office of the Surgeon General, 1997.

British Red Cross: The Family Reunion Department may be able to trace missing family members and can be contacted through local offices (in the phone book under B) or write to International Welfare Department, British Red Cross, 9 Grosvenor Crescent, London SW1X 7EJ.

Chemical and biological warfare: information is available online at *http://www.oneworld.org/ips2/mar98/iraq2.html*

HIV/AIDS: a list of specialist solicitors is available from the Terrence Higgins Trust (Tel: 0207 831 0330).

Immunization schedules for different countries are available online at *http://www11.who.int/vaccines/globalsummary/Immunization/CountryProfileSelect.cfm.*

Refugee Council Panel of Advisers for Unaccompanied Refugee Children: offers support to unaccompanied children under the age of 18 when they arrive and people aged 18–21 years who are the main carers for younger siblings (240–250 Ferndale Road, London SW9 8BB Tel: 0207 582 4947).

Index

Printed in the United Kingdom
by Lightning Source UK Ltd.
109227UKS00001B/235

. 9 780198 515739